Praise for *Glimpses of Raja Yoga*

Despite yoga's popularity, many students are unaware of the depth of its philosophy, its roots, and its applications. Vimala Thakar offers a remedy in *Glimpses of Raja Yoga: An Introduction to Patanjali's Yoga Sutras*. With scrupulous attention to language, she presents a clear interpretation of yoga's timeless principles in ways that inspire and encourage. A careful reading will provide a better understanding of the basic concepts of yoga philosophy and, more important, help you to live your understanding.

—Judith Hanson Lasater, Ph.D, P.T., author of
30 Essential Yoga Poses: For Beginning Students and Their Teachers

Glimpses of Raja Yoga

By Vimala Thakar

Blossoms of Friendship (2003)

Glimpses of Raja Yoga (2005)

glimpses of raja yoga

AN INTRODUCTION TO
PATANJALI'S YOGA SUTRAS

Vimala Thakar

YOGA WISDOM CLASSICS

Shambhala
Boulder 2005

Shambhala Publications, Inc.
2129 13th Street
Boulder, Colorado 80302
www.shambhala.com
A Rodmell Press book

First edition (1991) and second edition (1998) published by Vimal Prakashan Trust, Ahmedabad, India.

Printed in the United States of America

Shambhala Publications makes every effort to print on acid-free, recycled paper.

Shambhala Publications is distributed worldwide by Penguin Random House, Inc., and its subsidiaries.

Editor: Kaiser Irani
Series Editor: Donald Moyer
Copy Editor: Katherine L. Kaiser
Sanskrit Consultant: Robert Raddock
Cover and Book Designer: Gopa & Ted2, Inc.
Author Photograph: Courtesy of What Is Enlightenment?
Indexer: Ty Koontz
Production Editor: Linda Cogozzo

Text set in Bembo

Library of Congress Cataloging-in-Publication Data

Thakar, Vimala.
Glimpses of raja yoga: an introduction to Patanjali's Yoga sutras/Vimala Thakar; [editor, Kaiser Irani].—1st North American pbk. ed.
p. cm.—(Yoga wisdom classics)
Previous ed.: 2nd ed. Ahmedabad, India: Vimal Prakashan Trust, 1998.
ISBN 978-1-930485-07-5 (pbk.: alk. paper)
1. Yoga, Rāja. 2. Patañjali Yogasūtra. I. Irani, Kaiser. II. Title. III. Series.
BL1238.56.R35T43 2005
181'.452—dc22
2004021799

Contents

Preface

At the request of friends who are yoga teachers in Italy, Vimalaji gave a series of talks and answered a number of questions on Patanjali's Raja Yoga, in Italy in 1989.

Outside India, Vimalaji has never spoken about yoga or about the Upanishads with non-Indians. It was in March 1989 when some friends from Italy came over to Mount Abu and spent ten days studying Ishavasya Upanishad, that Vimalaji first spoke about the Upanishads, and after Ishavasya Upanishad, in August 1989 Vimalaji spoke about Raja Yoga in Italy.

As such talks on the ancient teachings of Indian sages and rishis are being published for the first time in English, we would like to draw the attention of all our readers, inquirers, and students of yoga to the fact that during the talks Vimalaji clarified that what was being said was about Patanjali Yoga. "Vimala is not sitting here to talk about her understanding of life. She is sitting here as a teacher would sit in a class to talk about Raja Yoga, which is a philosophy of Patanjali. So with great respect I share my understanding of those aphorisms."

As these dialogues were a response to questions on different sutras, they were in no way a complete study of the Yoga Sutras. In 1996 there was a request from the Yoga teachers of Europe for an in-depth study of Patanjali's Yoga Sutras. Vimalaji accepted their request and in September 1996 for two weeks Vimalaji took up the study of Patanjali's Raja Yoga. We are happy to inform our readers that a book has now been published based on those dialogues titled *Yoga Beyond Meditation*.

—Kaiser Irani
Editor

CHAPTER ONE

The Foundation of the Science of Raja Yoga

During this one week that we are together, discourses will not be given, but there will be a very intimate sharing about Raja Yoga, which is a holistic way of living. As you consider yourself to be students of yoga, Vimala considers herself a student of the holistic way of living, so we are going to share, sitting in a class, as it were, and talk things over, as intimately as possible.

Let us lay the foundation for our one-week inquiry in this, our first morning session. I'm afraid I will be obliged to use a number of Sanskrit terms. One would like to avoid using them, as far as possible, but certain terms would not be avoidable. We have to look at them and understand them before we proceed with our study of Raja Yoga.

Yoga as a way of living was discovered in India thousands and thousands of years ago. It is not a philosophy or a science that came into existence only in 553 B.C., when Patanjali codified the way of living into certain sutras. The study of the sutras by themselves—the words, their literal meaning—is an introduction to yoga, but the aphorisms, or the sutras, of Patanjali do not constitute the whole of yoga.

In order to understand Patanjali, we will have to go back into Vedic history or, rather, the history of Vedic culture in India. In order to lay the foundation of inquiry, you will have to get acquainted with the culture in which Patanjali could write down those aphorisms. Discoveries have their roots in culture. They are not born in the emptiness or void, but are rather the by-products of a collective way of living. Long before Patanjali was born, the Vedas were written. Even if you accept the European version of Indian history, the Vedas were written ten thousand years ago. According to the Chinese and the Indian historians, the Vedas go back fifteen thousand years.

History of the Vedic Period

The word *veda* is derived from the root *vid. Vid* is "to know"—*vid, veda, vedānta. Vedānta* is "the ending of knowledge." *Veda* is "the product of knowledge." *Vid* is to know, to acquire information about cosmic life, to investigate through observation, exploration, experimentation and then to write down the truth that has been verified by oneself in the laboratory of one's life.

I would like your attention to be drawn to this point, that in the Vedas, the words that were written are communications of verified truths by the rishis or the sages (by whatever means they had for verification) in the laboratory of their physical and psychological lives. They investigated, explored, experimented and in the laboratory of relationships the truths were verified, because the validity of truth can be discovered only in the movement of relationships. If the truths do not stand valid or stand the test of living them in the actual movement of relationship, then the truths are nothing but theories gathered intellectually, stored in memory, and repeated like philosophies.

The Vedas are not volumes of philosophy—they are freely verbalized and written-down communications of the verified truth. That is the first thing one would like to point out about the Vedic culture and the Vedas. The Rig Veda, Yajur Veda, Sama Veda, Atharva Veda were verbally communicated. They had no paper or printing press, so they would take the bark of a tree and write on it. The oldest copies of the Vedas are still on these barks of trees. The name of the tree was *bhuja* and the bark was called *bhoja*. On the *bhoja patra*—the bark of the bhuja tree—the Vedas were written.

Rishis

The Vedas are a collection of communications of verified truths, and these truths are about the origin of the cosmos and cosmic life. They are about the nature of interrelationships among the things and beings that inhabit the cosmos, the nature of nonhuman and human species. They are about biology, physiology, psychology, sexology, genetic engineering, music, dance, drama, poetry, to mention only a few. There is not a single aspect of life—human as well as nonhuman—that was not investigated by those ancient sages who were called rishis. The Sanskrit word for a sage was *ṛṣi*.

The person was called a rishi because the word *ṛṣi* is derived from the Sanskrit root that implied "to perceive." A rishi is an individual whose perceptions are purified.

In English you call such a person a sage, but the word *sage* does not have the nuances contained in the word *ṛṣi*. *Ṛṣi* means purified perception, austerity to live the perception as it has taken place, and the capacity to teach if students come to them. A rishi must have these three things:

- Purified perception *(ṛṣyo mantradṛṣṭāro)*. They perceive. They can perceive the sound and the quality of sound, they can perceive light and the constituent principles of light, they can perceive even where perceptions are subtle, fine, purified.
- The strength of austerity or, rather, the strength to dedicate one's life to the living of truth. You might perceive the truth but not live it. Then you cannot be called a rishi. The living is the test of the understanding. Knowledge for the sake of knowledge, knowledge for the sake of scholarship, knowledge for propagation of theories—all were meaningless in the Vedic period. So they required the discipline, the austerity, to live those truths, to dedicate their lives to living the truths.
- The capacity to communicate. If the student came to learn, then you can take the role of a teacher and communicate.

These three attributes enable a person to be called a rishi or a sage.

Ṛṣi Saṃskṛti

The Vedas were written by rishis and they lived in forests. The period of Vedic culture is called *ṛṣi saṃskṛti*—the culture of rishis. The rishis always lived in the forest, so in Indian history you might find the phrase *āraṇyaka saṃskṛti* —forest culture. *Araṇya* is the word for "forest" and *saṃskṛti* means "culture." Rishis were living in the *araṇya* writing down the Vedas, so it was called *āraṇyaka saṃskṛti.* Some of the Vedas are called *Āraṇyakas,* that is to say, the discovery of truth that took place in the forest.

Saṃskṛti is the Sanskrit word used for "culture." Civilization is the advance of science and technology, and culture is the conditioning of the consciousness. The process through which the conditioning of consciousness takes place is called culture or a culture-building activity. Civilization refers to the outer, to the external, and, to some extent, even to the physical. But in culture you are referring to the inner, and how you mold, shape, regulate the quality of consciousness among individuals and among groups of individuals. In Sanskrit the word is *saṃskṛti.*

Saṃskṛti is the result of conditionings. Now please do see with me that the word *conditioning* that I am using has a special psychological connotation in the Western world. The word *conditioning* means "limitation," and when you say, "This is my conditioning," you refer to your limitations, and sometimes the word is used in a derogatory sense. But the Sanskrit words *saṃskāra, saṃskāram,* and *saṃskṛti* do not mean limiting the content. The purpose is not to limit the content. The purpose is not to limit, but to mold and shape, for example, to mold and regulate the animal instincts in the human being. Why should they be regulated or controlled or molded? They should be regulated, controlled, or molded so that they do not become obstacles or hurdles in the expression of something that human beings have more than animals have. In order to help the expression, hurdles or obstacles have to be removed or they have to be channeled. Human instincts have to be channeled, they have to be shaped and regulated so that the Divinity, the inexhaustible creativity, the potential creativity in human beings can express itself in daily living. *Saṃskāra* is not regarded as a bondage or means of limitation, but as a help for the expression of the being, as a help for manifesting the content of being.

Saṃskṛti is the result of such collective efforts at regulating, molding, shaping, and channeling the animal instincts, the roughness, the cruelty, so that the human being becomes a *mānava saṃskṛta*—a cultured human being. Culture is the process of helping the Divinity within to manifest itself at every level of life—physical, verbal, psychological. In the movement of relationship it is the content of Divinity that has to be expressed, it is the content of wholeness that has to be expressed. Whatever prevents the wholeness from manifesting would be looked upon as an obstacle, and whatever helps the wholeness to manifest, to get reflected, to express itself would be looked upon as *saṃskṛti,* or cultured.

The Vedas were written by the rishis living in the forests developing ways of living, so that the potential creativity which human beings share with the cosmos smoothly manifests itself at the physical, the verbal, and the psychological level. The Vedas are equal to *ṛṣi saṃskṛti,* the culture of the sages.

Kṛṣi Saṃskṛti

In order to see the background, I will proceed to look at another aspect, because this Vedic culture, or *ṛṣi saṃskṛti,* required a social background and that social background was agriculture. Agriculture in Sanskrit is called *kṛṣi.* The first was *ṛṣi* and rishi culture, and the second was *kṛṣi* and krishi culture. *Kṛṣi* is "to till the land." The forest cultures were accompanied by agriculture; they were in harmony with each other. The land was tilled. It was not treated as an industry, and the relationship with the land was not one of getting input from the land and output from the land. It was not looked upon as a factory or industry. Commercialization—all these things were not known. I'm trying to persuade you to come back with me five thousand years to a human culture where commercialization of life was not even dreamed of. There was reverence for life, there was gratefulness for life.

The rishis and their culture were accompanied by farmers and their farms. Forest culture and farm culture. If you don't understand these two together, we are not going to get at the essence of Raja Yoga. When you turn to the aphorisms, the words will remain empty words, with some dictionary meaning, unrelated to our food, to our diet, to our psychology, to our behavior. They will remain only theories. An intellectual study of theories never leads to a transformation of your being and your life. Whatever one studies has to be correlated to one's way of living. Knowledge unrelated to your way of living has no value. As soon as knowledge is related to your act of living, correlated to everything—from the moment of birth to the moment of death—when it gets correlated to every activity, then knowledge gets converted into understanding. It becomes the substance of your being, and then transformation is a by-product of the conversion of the substance of your being. You do not have to work for it. Mutation, transformation, psychic revolution are not intellectual exercises, they are not emotional cultivation—they are the by-product, a natural logical consequence of something much deeper.

So the forest culture in the Vedic days was accompanied by farm culture. Rishi culture and krishi culture. The land was tilled with love and reverence, with gratefulness, so that people could grow grains, cereals, vegetables, fruits, etc.

There used to be in those days what you call kings or princes who took care of the forests or farms. They were called in Sanskrit *nṛpati*. *Pati* is "a protector" and *nṛ* means "human being." Protector of human beings. The responsibility of the kings was to protect the rishis and the farmers. The farmers were the producers of the basic necessities of life, and the rishis, the givers of the light of understanding. These three were working intelligently, in cooperation with one another. There was a holistic way of living. If this had not existed, I wonder if the Yoga Sutras could have been written or, for that matter, whether any other branch of yoga—Mantra Yoga, Tantra Yoga—could have resulted at all. Because these discoveries, requiring the dedication of generations, also required a security, a stability—economic stability and political security, as you call them today. I would say psychological security and physical security is required, so that one can relax and dedicate oneself. These rishis had dedicated their lives to the discoveries of truth, to the discoveries of the nature of Ultimate Reality. They were privileged to dedicate their lives. They could convert their bodies and their lives into laboratories because the farmers were there to feed them and the *nṛpati* was there to protect them. They did not have to work. Please take into consideration this context of life, this harmonious, holistic living.

Āśrama Saṃskṛti

How did the teaching of the rishis, the Vedas, the Upanishads, the Aranyakas, the Samhitas, the Brahmanas, the Vyakaras, etc., how did it travel downward from 5,000 years back, right to the twenty-first century? It is beautiful the way the rishis lived there in the forests with their families. Their doors were open twenty-four hours to anyone who wanted to come and learn from them; that is why their homes were called *āśrama*. *Śram* is "exhaustion"—physical, psychological. It is a place, in other words, where you relax. *Āśrama* is a place of total relaxation, where relaxation is a way of living or the way of living is relaxed, whichever way you like to put it.

The homes of the rishis were like universities. Whoever wanted to go and study could approach the rishi and say, "I would like to come and study with you." Then the students had to live in the forests with those sages as members of their family and share all the work—cutting the wood, cooking the meals, washing the utensils, etc. Living and learning were woven together. I'm trying to share with you how the holistic way was holistic in every detail. Today education is a profession. Teaching is a profession, and for those who go to school or college, learning is a part-time thing. You pay money for it and you get taught, you get a degree, so that you get a job, and so on. The learning was not a profession nor was teaching a profession. The students and the teachers lived together. The learners and those who had learned before them, they came together and lived together and learned together.

When living and learning get divorced from each other, when learning loses its co-relation with living, then I think people become knowledgeable, but they understand very little because the very act of learning is not co-related to living. In the Vedic period, learning was a part of living, living was a movement of learning and communicating.

In Sanskrit, the word used for "teaching" is *ācārya*. *Ācāra* means "your behavior," *ācārya* is "one in whose behavior all his understanding is manifested effortlessly." *Ācāra*, or the behavior, is the test of your understanding. The criterion or norm of testing whether the teacher was good or not was his behavior—his relationship with his wife, with the students who came to learn, with the land while working on the farm or in the forest.

The students came and the rishis taught. The spoken word was received. There were no books, no writing notes. You had to receive very deeply with the wholeness of your being. When you have notebooks, you write down notes. When you have cassettes, you don't even take notes—you sit before the cassettes and you listen to them. Everything is so abstract now—listening is no more the movement of your whole being. Our life today is a fragmented way of living. It is a compartmentalized way of living, and in order to move toward the holistic way of living, we will have to meet these challenges. We cannot go back to the farm culture, we cannot go back to the Vedic culture, but out of the complications of the modern industrialized world and the cultural and spiritual crisis it has created for us, we will have to find a holistic way of living. Moving out of this fragmentation and developing a holistic way in the context of the twenty-first century. Do you see the challenge that is facing us? Otherwise, I would not be talking about yoga to you.

If human beings five thousand years ago had the genius to live holistically, then I think human beings today also can have the same genius to carve out a holistic way of living and proceed from the twentieth century to the twenty-first century. The twentieth century has been the bloodiest, the most murderous, century in history. Let the twenty-first be a century of creativity. The nineteenth and twentieth centuries were ones of specialization, compartmentalization, and fragmentation on race, on religion, on nationality, and so on. Let the twenty-first century be a century of discovering a holistic way of living, a holistic diet, holistic medicine, holistic exercises, holistic relationships—wholeness as the content of consciousness—a holistic perspective on life. That is the challenge waiting for us, and I think Raja Yoga points a way to the possibility of a holistic century.

Students came and started living with the teacher for twenty-four hours a day, exposed to the searchlight of intimacy. Small children and adults were watching, were observing the teacher in his privacy, in his classes—everywhere. Whatever is valid after having been exposed to the intimacy of living together has some value in life. Otherwise, you will be speaking one thing and living in quite a contradictory way. As we said a few minutes ago, living is the test of understanding, and the movement of understanding is the test of the quality of your consciousness. Whatever your consciousness is, it is bound to be expressed in relationship. You can't say, "I have peace," and in relationship get disturbed, perturbed, imbalanced every second hour.

The teachings were received with the wholeness of being. They sprang from the wholeness of being and were received with the wholeness of being. Through the centuries the Vedas were not written down, but for thousands and thousands of years they were just received, lived, communicated, like a river flowing.

If these points have been sufficiently clear as the background of yoga, let us proceed. All the Upanishads are in the form of dialogue between the teacher and the student. There are hundreds of such Upanishads, and on the basis of these Upanishads is the flowering of the Vedas. After the period of the Upanishads comes the period of codifying and putting them scientifically in the form of treatise or thesis. Sankhya, Yoga, Nyaya, Vaisheshika, Purva Mimamsa, Uttar Mimamsa—the six schools of philosophy. You get first the five Vedas, then the five hundred Upanishads, then you get the six systems of Indian philosophy, among which you get Yoga as the second school of philosophy. First comes Sankhya and then comes Yoga, third comes Nyaya, or logic, then the Vaisheshika, the analysis of matter, then Purva Mimamsa, and Uttar Mimamsa, or Vedanta, the ending of knowledge. The six systems of Indian philosophy came after the period of the Upanishads. I could go into details with you about the Upanishadic period also, but it is not necessary.

The details about the history of the Vedic period were necessary, because they laid the foundation of a holistic perspective, for they claimed that wholeness can be the content of consciousness. The claim of the Yoga Sutras of Patanjali, the claim of Vedanta, is uniquely this: that the content of consciousness—thought, emotion—can be an organic wholeness. The *vṛtti* need not be oscillating all the time—the content of consciousness can be an organic wholeness. As there is an organic wholeness in the cosmos of the human consciousness, the content can also be an organic wholeness, which could be called no-thing-ness or all-thingness—so this foundation was necessary.

Yoga

Let us refer today to the word *yoga.* Yoga indicates a science and the art of blending that which has been separated, that which has been individuated. Yoga is the science and the art of helping the individual to merge back into a nonindividuated wholeness. That which has been separated is helped to come back, to join together, and blend into the indivisible, nonfragmentable wholeness.

Yuj, yujyate. Yuj is "to combine, to join, to blend." It has a number of meanings, but the root is *yuj,* from which the word *yoga* is formed.

The science of yoga became a science, an art of joining, combining, blending that which was separated, fragmented, individuated. The cosmos is an emergence of creative energies and their interactions, in which we find there is also what you call death, which is a merging back of the expressions of these energies. I don't know how else to put it.

There is inexhaustible creative energy that is Life. This inexhaustible creative energy manifests itself in the form of a cosmos, infinite universes. It is an emergence, a manifestation, and after some time the expressions merge back. Life, emergence, merging back. There is not life—creation and destruction. There is nothing like destruction in nature, in cosmic Life. In the realm and in the orbit of intelligence, there is nothing like destruction or death. There is only emergence and merging back—a cyclic movement, a circular movement, a holistic movement of emergence and merging back, emergence and merging back.

The science of yoga itself flowered into many branches. So those who studied sound metaphysics, they brought forth Mantra Yoga. Those who studied the energies and energy centers in the human body with special emphasis on sex energy, they developed Tantra Yoga. Those who studied the art of merging energies, they developed Laya Yoga. Those who concentrated on the fire principle and the breath in the body, they developed Hatha Yoga. Those who specialized in using action as the way of going back to the root of life, they developed Karma Yoga. Those who used devotion as a path for getting back to the root of life, they developed Bhakti Yoga. The science of yoga flowered into so many branches, but you come to the trunk of the tree and that is Raja Yoga.

Raja Yoga

In Raja Yoga there is no specialization only on sound, only on breath, only on physical postures, only on devotion, or only on *jñana,* or knowledge. Instead, it is a holistic path. When you go through Ashtanga Yoga, you go through all the postures and pranayama not separately, but when you are doing things you are aware of the whole. In the movement of action you are aware of the movement of the breath, you are aware of the glandular, the muscular, the neurological movement. The physical, the verbal, the psychic—they are all woven together. Raja Yoga is the culmination of these different branches of yoga that have specialized in one or two directions. Raja Yoga is not a specialization in one direction. In its compass it takes the whole life—individual and collective; physical, verbal, and psychic; human and cosmic; birth and death. *Rāja* literally means "the prince." Raja Yoga is the prince of yoga.

This introductory meeting was aimed at laying the foundation. Before we turn to Raja Yoga, we must be aware that it had the background of the rishi culture, which was interested in a holistic perspective of life and manifesting wholeness as the content of consciousness. If these investigations, experimentations, explorations of hard work in the laboratory of the human body and brain had not taken place, we would not have inherited from the Vedas, the Upanishads, and the rishis like Patanjali what they have got to tell us.

Discoveries of the Vedic Period

The first thing that the science of yoga tells us is that there is nothing inanimate in life. Life is not a totality that has been artificially created by assembling parts and putting them together. It is not an integrated totality of parts put together. Earth, water, fire, air were not put together and then the cosmos was created. It is a homogeneous, self-generated, self-sustained organic wholeness.

Look at this discovery made thousands of years ago! These people, through their investigations, their experimentations on their bodies, they arrived at this truth. This basic truth is one that we have to learn and incorporate into our way of living, that the whole cosmos is an organism. The planet Earth is a living organism vibrating with Life. Life permeates every body. Life permeates everything. Do not call the Earth a thing, do not call a tree, a mountain, or a river a thing. They are beings. You know, the whole cosmos is a living organism, and it has parts like the human body has parts—hands, feet, eyes, nose, etc. The trees, the mountains, the oceans, the rivers, the animals, birds, and human beings—they are all interrelated in a very intelligent way. Call it a mysterious way.

So there is:

- Organic wholeness of Life
- Interrelatedness of every being, of every expression of Life
- An intelligent harmony permeating the whole cosmos.

These were the three discoveries of the Vedic and the Upanishadic period, upon which the science of Raja Yoga is based.

CHAPTER TWO

The Dimension of Silence

Yogaś-citta-vṛtti-nirodhaḥ (I.2)

Question: If the calming of the mind is ultimately an involuntary process, how important is the practice of sitting in Silence—a voluntary practice—in reaching the state of consciousness described in Patanjali's sutra *yogaś-citta-vṛtti-nirodhaḥ?*

Our modern way of living ignores the dimension of Silence, or motionlessness; Silence, or sound-freeness; Silence, or thought-freeness. This dimension of consciousness is complete freedom from the movement of thoughts, complete freedom from sound or verbalization, and also complete freedom from the movement of relationships. Life is a movement of sound and speech as well as the magnificence of Silence. Life is a dance of the interaction of energies, a movement of innumerable energies as well as the grandeur of motionlessness, or stillness.

This second dimension is ignored by modern civilization. In education, at home, through social compulsion, human beings are trained in thinking, knowing, experiencing, organizing relationships, standardizing patterns of reaction, playing around with physical, verbal, psychological movements. The dimension of movement is emphasized and the other is ignored. So we have the necessity of self-education. We have to learn to educate ourselves for growing into the dimension of stillness, of motionlessness, of sound-freeness, of thought-freeness, and of aloneness.

When we sit in Silence, first we begin by educating the body in steadiness. The body is moving the whole day—neurologically, chemically.

There are movements outside the body like sitting, standing, walking, running, etc., and there are inner movements also. So constant movement is going on. When we come to sit down, we learn to steady the body. You put the body in a posture which is convenient, agreeable, enjoyable to the body and persuade it to be steady for half an hour. This is education—not a technique, not a method. You have to help the body, you have to educate the body. This is an educational process if you would like to call it that.

And then you close your eyes, so that the eyes do not touch any matter outside the body, any object outside the body. Because as soon as the eyes see the object, the memory throws back the name of the object, the memory throws back your attachment to the object, your likes, your dislikes, your differences, your prejudices, your value judgments—so the movement begins. As we want to help the brain to be steady, to be motionless, to be still, we close the eyes—that also is a help. Once you have tasted the nectar of Silence, then whether your eyes are open or closed, it does not make any difference. Once you have tasted the nectar of that dimension, then it does not matter whether you are sitting in a room or working in an office or the kitchen or talking to people. The quality of aloneness, the quality of motionlessness, the quality of thought-freeness does not get affected by physical or verbal movement.

Thirdly, you abstain from speaking. Our modern way of living requires verbalization most of the time. Speaking aloud to other people. As we have to work for eight hours a day at some job, verbalization is necessary, externally speaking to people is necessary. And if that is not done, then you do it internally—chattering to yourself. We have been trained in schools and colleges, the brain has been trained to think, to acquire and organize information, to compare and evaluate it, that is to say, make a judgment about it. We are conditioned by society, by religion to accept it as good or to reject it as not good. These conditionings are imprinted in what you call the brain, so the brain is all the time busy. Instead of using thought, knowledge, the capacity to imagine, the faculty of memory only when it is necessary, as a handy instrument, we have become addicted to the movement of knowledge within us, to the movement of comparison, evaluation within us, to the movement of likes and dislikes within us. The movement goes on within ourselves throughout the day, and some people do it even when they are sleeping throughout their dreams. The activity goes on. When you sit in Silence you are educating the brain to be free of that incessant movement of knowing, experiencing, accepting, rejecting. Let the brain be free of those activities.

Please do see what learning to sit in Silence implies. If you have learned, and then you sit in Silence, you do it for the joy of it, because now it is no longer necessary, it has become a way of living. When you spend eight hours in bed and sleep every night, do you practice sleep? Do you say that we practice sleep? You just sleep. That becomes the content of life and living. In the same way, Silence, the dimension of thought-free consciousness, sound-free consciousness, relationship-free consciousness becomes the dimension in which you live. That is one aspect of Silence.

If you would take the journey with me, let us look at another aspect of this dimension of Silence. I hope you are aware, as students of yoga, that Raja Yoga is not only yama, niyama, asana, pranayama—they are important parts of it, but they are a fraction of it, just a part of Raja Yoga. Raja Yoga is much wider, the horizons are much wider than that of Hatha Yoga or that given to you in Hatha Yoga Pradipika or in Gheranda Samhita. Raja Yoga is much wider, and being students of yoga, I hope you will accompany me and look at the dimension of Silence from a different angle.

Have you noticed that all knowledge is on the ideational plane? Knowledge consists of thought, and thought is built up through words and their order. Knowledge is nothing but ideas, concepts, theories, evaluations. All knowledge is ideational. The life by which we are surrounded, the life of which we are born, is thought-free, is measurement-free, is idea-free. You create an idea of time and you live in the framework of time—of hours, days, years, centuries. The eternity of time has nothing to do with your idea of time. Time is an idea that mankind builds up for the convenience of relationship. They want to live together and they must have a measurement. You measure space by kilometers, but the infinity of space is free of all your measurements of kilometers or miles.

We are born of cosmic life, we are born of the wholeness of cosmic life, where there are no ideas, no measurements, no thoughts. The Divinity is absolutely free of the word *God*, the word *God* is not the content of Divinity. It existed before mankind came to the globe, inhabited the planet, and it shall remain there.

So what we call knowledge, what we call thought, which is the content, the substance of our consciousness, is on the ideational level. It is upon the level of ideas, not the Reality. I wonder if you have noticed the difference between the Reality of Life and the ideational state that mankind has created which we call culture, philosophy, theology? Let us take an example. Imagine we are standing on a river bank. The word *river* is in the human brain; outside, there is a curvature of land and water flowing through it. That is all. As an objective fact, there is the curvature of land and water flowing, but the combination has been called by the human brain a *river.* Do you understand *river* is an idea that exists in our brains only? The flowing waters and the curvature of the land may be called objective reality, but Reality is free of the word *river.*

On the perceptual, objective level, mankind has created an ideational, subjective perception. So we live simultaneously on the material plane surrounded by Life, which is idea-free, which is concept-free. On the conceptual, ideational level, these concepts and ideas are necessary. We have used them for centuries and we shall have to use them as long as we live in society and share life. So we have to coin words, constitute language, have grammar, syntax, phonetics, linguistics, semantics—that is how we live. Throughout the day, you and I, we have to move on the ideational level, using words, thoughts, ideas, measurements. Even the ego, the self is an idea. We are required to distinguish between persons and forms, so we gave them names and identified them, and created an idea about the self, the "Me." The I-ness in consciousness is an idea; we have to use it.

I'm not going into the details of this ideational dimension. We have to live in it, but there is Life that is entirely free of all this—the I-ness, the Me-ness, the psychological time.

When we sit in Silence and put ourselves in a state of nonexperiencing, nonknowing, nondoing, nonspeaking, we are moving away from the ideational dimension, the artificially structured dimension (which is necessary for social life) and plunging into the Real. Silence is like taking a plunge into knowledge-free Reality. The whole thought structure and its movement has gone into abeyance, and we have set ourselves free of it, as if we have jumped out of the stream of knowledge.

So this is the second importance of educating ourselves to be in the dimension of Silence—to be free of the clutches of knowledge, to be free of the clutches of the ideational, the conceptual world.

Do you know what aloneness is? Aloneness is being free of the movement of thought. Aloneness is being free of the movement of verbalization. That is relaxation, not only stretching your hands and feet and lying down in *śavāsana. Śavāsana* can give physical relaxation, but we are talking about something deeper than physical relaxation. This is psychic relaxation. To be completely free of thoughts, measurements, concepts, judgments, reactions.

The holiness, the sacredness of Life is in this dimension of Reality. No idea or thought can be sacred. By creating compulsions for ourselves to use the thought, the knowledge, we have moved away from the sacredness of Life, we have moved away from nature. That is what the ecologists tell us. They want you to see the sanctity of nature, to respect it, but we are taking it one step further than the ecologists—we are saying that the Reality that is not touched by thought is sacred, is holy.

In your daily living, when you spend some time in the sanctity of that Reality, in that wholeness, then you have moved away from all fragmentations, distinctions, compartmentalizations, and you are back at the source of your wholeness and the source of wholeness around you. That is learning to be in Silence. Not only sitting down still, closing your eyes, and not speaking by the mouth—that is external—that is not the essence. The essence is quite different. Thus when you are in the Real, with the Real, that is to say, with Reality untouched by thought, untouched by knowledge, when you are there, then you are in the state of *yogaś-citta-vṛtti-nirodhaḥ*. When the thought movement *(vṛtti)* is not there, obviously no emotions, no sentiments are there.

In the educational period, that state remains with you when you are sitting in Silence, and when the educational period is over, you live in that knowledge-free content of consciousness, you live in that total relaxation of aloneness and use the handy instrument of knowledge only if and when it is necessary.

So an alternative way of living, an alternative human culture can come into existence through the study of Raja Yoga.

CHAPTER THREE

The Yamas 1

Ahiṃsā-satya-asteya-brahmacarya-aparigrahā yamāḥ (II.30)

Question: Please speak to us about the yamas and niyamas.

Question: Given our different cultural upbringing, it is difficult for us in the West to understand the meaning of *brahmacarya*. Can you explain to us your interpretation of *brahmacarya*?

Ahiṃsā

When you are dedicated to an awareness of the wholeness of Life, to the interrelatedness of everything that you see in life, naturally your life becomes a dedication to *ahiṃsā,* or nonkilling, nonviolence. That becomes a value of your life, it becomes a demonstration that you do not hurt anyone intentionally, you do not want to destroy anything or anyone, you want to have an intelligent, cooperative, harmonious relationship.

Ahiṃsā is an intelligent, harmonious relationship. Harmony is the essence of nonviolence. It is not only nonkilling on the physical level. Supposing that a person does not kill and even takes vegetarian meals, but if he kills the hearts of people by his cruel, cold glances and destructive, abusive words, he is not a nonviolent person. If by behavior, by glances, by words you attack, invade the psyches of other people, you are not a nonviolent person. You may not kill physically, but you are killing psychologically, you are hurting by eyes, you are hurting by words.

When you are aware of the organic wholeness of Life and the interrelatedness of everything in Life, naturally there is an urge to live harmoniously with everything and every being. You move intelligently so that there is a harmony with the human species, with nonhuman species, harmony with the mountains, rivers, oceans, trees, and birds. Not to use anything or not to use anyone as an instrument of your sensual pleasure. You don't use sex or sexual relationships as a means of escape from freedom or as an outlet for your aggressive desires. You don't run toward a sex relationship to escape from fear.

As *ahiṃsā* or a harmonious, intelligent, cooperative life becomes a demonstration of your Raja Yoga, *brahmacarya* also becomes a demonstration of the awareness that Life is one, Life is unity, Life is interrelationship.

Satya

It seems to me that Raja Yoga is pointing a way toward a human culture and human society where nonkilling, nonstealing, truthfulness, etc., would be the values of life. Truthfulness means we are dedicated to the truth we perceive, to the truth we understand. So when you communicate through words, you communicate that truth without underrating, overrating it, without using superlative degrees, without putting your excessive feelings in it. You say, you communicate as you have seen it.

Truthfulness is harmony with the fact, harmony with the motive. If you hide your motivation, you are not truthful. If you have not done something and you pretend you have done something, then you have walked away from truthfulness. It is a psychophysical, harmonious way.

Our lives are maladjusted, both to our inner motivations and the outer facts. Therefore there is a necessity to say, "Let there be truthfulness." If there were no maladjustment in verbalization, it would not be necessary to say that truthfulness should be a value, but because there is so much maladjustment, because we go on speaking lies, exaggerating things, pretending to be what we are not, being hypocrites, that education in verbal truthfulness, psychic truthfulness becomes a necessity.

The yamas do not give you a code of conduct—they give you a perspective on life, an evaluation of life, they give you an attitude toward life. I hope you see the difference. They give you guidelines for life, because, after all, Raja Yoga is a transformation of the perspective on life—from a fragmentary, compartmental perspective to a holistic perspective. It is a transformation in the content of consciousness. Instead of being always filled with thought and knowledge, it is now in the excellence of emptiness. So please do not look upon the yamas as giving you a rigid code of conduct.

The niyamas are quite different from the yamas. The niyamas are relative values. The yamas are universal. Your cultural differences do not affect the necessity for every human being to observe the yamas. They are relevant both to the East and the West—whether it is *brahmacarya,* whether it is *ahiṃsā,* whether it is *satya.*

Asteya

Let us look at the word *asteya,* which is translated in English commentaries as "nonstealing." What does that mean? You and I will not go stealing things from one another's houses or offices. What is the relevance of the word *asteya,* nonstealing? What does the word *nonstealing* imply as a yama?

Just to call it nonstealing, not being a thief, would be a very cheap rendering of something very precious communicated by Patanjali. To accept things of personal use for which you have not worked—physically, mentally, intellectually. To go on accepting things like unearned income, life securities, unemployment doles that are given by the governments and for which you have not worked. I do not know about Europe, but they do provide unemployment doles in the U.S.A., in Australia. To have the austerity not to have an inclination, wish, or expectation—verbalized or unverbalized—to get anything for which one has not worked.

Do you see the importance of the quality of consciousness that would feel it below its dignity to receive anything, to accept anything for which one has not worked? Do you see the importance of this yama when we modern human beings and our societies, our governments, our administrations are suffering from the cancerous disease of corruption? What is corruption? Corruption is to take money for which you don't work. You grab money without working for it, you want to have a profit much more than the ratio of the profit allows you. Do you see the roots of corruption, the source of corruption is in the quality of human consciousness that does not consider it is below its dignity, below its self-respect to receive anything from anyone—individually or collectively—for which one has not worked, physically or psychologically?

I do not know if the Marxists or the Communists ever understood *asteya,* but when Marx or Engels or Lenin talked about a society in which you take from everyone according to his capacity and you give to everyone according to his needs, without their knowing it, they were referring to the value of *asteya.*

Brahmacharya

Brahman is a Sanskrit word, and the root meaning of the word *Brahman* is "that which contains an inexhaustible potential of creativity." *Brahman* is a name given to the Ultimate Reality by the Vedas because it is inexhaustible creativity. For millions and billions of years, Life has been manifesting, the manifestations have been merging back into formlessness, but the dance of emergence of forms and merging back of forms into the formlessness goes on. So the name *Brahman* was given to unnameableness of inexhaustible Creativity.

Brahman is not a god, a goddess, it is only all-permeating Supreme Intelligence, because creativity is the characteristic of Intelligence.

The other part of the word *brahmacarya* is *acarya.* The word *carya* is derived from the root *car*—"to walk, to move, to live." *Caraiveti, caraiveti, caraiveti*—"Be always moving, be always moving, keep moving," the ancient sages used to say. "Never get static, never be idle, be on the move, be on the move, be creative." That is what the teacher would tell the student, when the student after his education returned to his home from the place of the teacher.

Carya means "the way of living." *Brahmacarya* is the way of living in which you are always aware of the Divinity, of the Supreme Intelligence. *Brahmacarya* is living a life dedicated to the awareness of Divinity.

Brahmacarya is dedication to the understanding of Divinity. Understanding takes place only when you have perceived something, seen something.

Brahmacarya implies perception of Divinity, understanding the nature of Divinity, and living in the awareness of Divinity.

It is a triple dedication to the perception, to the understanding, and to the awareness. This is not my interpretation. I'm just giving to you the literal meaning of the word *brahmacarya*. That is why it is included as one of the yamas of Ashtanga Yoga.

Ahiṃsā-satya-asteya-brahmacarya-aparigrahā yamāḥ (II.30). These are the absolute values of human life. It is not a code of conduct. Unless there are some absolute values that cannot be bargained away and consciousness is rooted in those values, it seems to me that sane and healthy societies cannot come into existence.

Raja Yoga mentions some of the absolute values and the education of human beings in the perception of those values. *Brahmacarya*—dedication to the perception, understanding, and awareness of Divinity—is one of the yamas.

The word *brahmacarya* has been narrowed down to mean "celibacy." The meaning of the word *brahmacarya* got limited to "celibacy, continence, refraining from a sex life." But this is an interpretation imposed upon the word *bramhacarya* by commentators that you have come across in India for thousands of years. And when the books of Indian philosophy got translated into English or French or German, the word *brahmacarya* was translated as celibacy.

Celibacy is a very limited thing. Dedication to the awareness of Divinity, dedication to the understanding of Divinity can be possible even in married life. Married life or sexual relationship, if it is not distorted, if it is not compulsive sex, obsessive sexuality, if it is a normal, sane, healthy part of human life, then marriage is not an obstacle. It cannot be an obstacle or a hurdle to the dedication to the Truth of Life. This is how Vimala sees it. I am not referring to the commentators of the Upanishads or Yoga Sutras. In many of the Indian languages they will insist upon *brahmacarya* as not being married, refraining from sex relationship. For me, that is not only a secondary thing, an unessential thing, but I think it is a rather incorrect interpretation imposed upon that sacred word *brahmacarya*.

Aparigraha

Aparigraha has been translated by the commentators as "nonpossession." Now you have to possess things, you have to have a house, a room to live in, food and clothing. Patanjali would not be stupid enough to say you should not possess anything and go around in a loincloth, which was not the meaning.

You acquire food, clothing, a place to live in, you acquire provisions for health. You have to acquire these essentials, but after acquisition you also begin to own the things and possess them. Please do see that acquisition for utility and acquisition for possessiveness—these two have a different quality altogether.

Acquisition for utility—according to your needs, you acquire and you take care of them, but then there is a sensual pleasure in owning and possessing. Possessiveness becomes a quality of consciousness. You want to own and possess just for the fun of it, just for the joy of it. You want to own and possess not only material things, you want to own and possess human beings. Wife possessing the husband and husband possessing the wife, boyfriend possessing the girlfriend.

Possessiveness has exclusiveness, there is an attachment. When you acquire for utility, it is a sane way of living. You don't have to go begging, you don't become monks. You acquire knowledge, money, you have a family, children, you live as a blossoming, flowering human being. But to acquire and to use without attachment or exclusiveness, without beginning to enjoy possessing possessions just for the sake of possessing. Possessiveness becomes the dominating quality and attitude. Therefore in Raja Yoga, Patanjali says acquisition for utility but not the distortion, the perversion of possessiveness. A sense of belonging is healthy, but attachment, expecting exclusive loyalty, exclusive fidelity, that is morbid. It is a very fine distinction between a sense of belonging, of friendship and possessiveness, attachment obsession.

Patanjali is talking about a new content of consciousness when he talks about the yamas—*ahiṃsa, satya, asteya, brahmacarya, aparigraha*—which are universal values of Life, applicable to all human beings, irrespective of their regional, cultural, or language differences.

CHAPTER FOUR

The Yamas 2

Iti jāti-deśa-kāla-samaya-anavacchinnāḥ sārvabhaumā mahā-vratam (II.31)

We saw yesterday that *ahiṃsā* (nonviolence or nonkilling), *satya* (truthfulness), *asteya* (nonstealing), *brahmacarya* (dedication to the Divinity of Life), and *aparigraha* (nonpossessiveness) are described by Patanjali as yamas.

And while elaborating upon these yamas he says, *iti jāti-deśa-kāla-samaya-anavacchinnāḥ sārvabhaumā mahā-vratam*. These two aphorisms give us the complete version of what yamas are.

He says the yamas which were described in the earlier aphorism are universal—*sārvabhaumā*. These have universal applicability and they are supreme, because they describe the absolute values of Life. They do not require any modification, they are universally applicable in any and every country, at any and every time, because they are absolute values.

Why are they absolute values of Life, and why are they universally applicable at every time? Because Life as it was perceived by the sages and by Patanjali himself is a homogeneous wholeness where every expression is interrelated to every other. The mystery of this interrelatedness of Life, the all-permeating Intelligence that is Life and the homogeneity of Life, is not a totality of abstract theories put together or integrated together. It has a homogeneity—a self-generated, self-sustained, organic, interrelated wholeness. That was the perception of Life, of *brahman,* as the word was used.

It being so, these values of truthfulness, nonviolence, nonpossessiveness, dedication to the awareness of the Divinity of Life—they become absolute values. Please do see that Patanjali is not asking us just to believe in what he says, he would like us to purify our perceptions and see the truth as he has seen it.

So he calls them *sārvabhaumā* and one more word, a very important word, is used— *mahā-vratam*. I'm aware that those who translate these philosophies, the Upanishads, etc., into English, French, German, or any other non-Sanskrit language, they translate the word *vratam* as "vow." A vow is that which you have to take with an effort of the will, but to my mind that is an incorrect translation, whether it is done by a Vivekananda or a Max Muller. *Vratam* does not mean a vow intentionally, purposefully taken and followed or practiced. The word *vratam* is derived from the root *vrī, vrīyate. Vrīyate*—that root word in Sanskrit means "a choiceless acceptance out of understanding." When a girl marries a boy, she says, "I have fallen in love." Then there is no argumentation, they don't sit down and logically work out why they have fallen in love with each other. There is a resistance-free, choiceless acceptance of each other by the whole being—that is what love is. Love causes choiceless acceptance by the whole being. When there is no resistance from within, then it becomes a *vratam. Varaṇam prīyate. Varaṇam* and *vratam*. I cannot translate, I would love to give you the nuances of that beautiful word, which is generally used to describe marriages that take place—the fusion, the blending that take place—out of a choiceless acceptance. As in love, in *vratam* there is a choiceless acceptance. Once you understand the truth, once you see it and understand it, then there is no resistance from within, and there is a choiceless acceptance by your whole being of the truth that was perceived. So the choiceless acceptance of the truth that one has perceived and understood becomes a *vratam*. So in the way of living, these yamas—*ahiṃsā, satya, asteya,* etc.—get incorporated choicelessly, they do not need any effort of the will, they do not need any struggle. If there is resistance, if there is an imposition from outside, then it cannot be called a *vratam*. It is not a vow, it is not an imposition, it is not an imitation, a conformity. Please do see this—otherwise, the whole charm of the yamas would be lost upon us.

Once you see them as absolute truths, because of the organic wholeness of Life, the Intelligence, the sensitivity within you accepts those truths choicelessly. They become a way of living, they become incorporated into your way of living, which becomes a holistic way of living.

CHAPTER FIVE

The Niyamas

In this aphorism, Patanjali gives the niyamas: *śauca-santoṣa-tapaḥ-svādhyāya-īśvara-praṇidhānāni niyamāḥ* (II.32).

Śauca

Śauca is purification. Purity as a result of purification. Purity is the by-product of the process of purification.

Santoṣa

Santoṣa is a sense of contentment that arises when you do not compare yourself with others. As long as there is comparison, there cannot be contentment. It is a noncomparative, noncompetitive approach to oneself, to one's actions, to one's acquisitions, etc.

So *santoṣa* is contentment, born of a noncomparative perception of one's life.

Tapas

Tapas is austerity, not mortification. Generally they translate this word into English as "mortification," where you have to torture the body, you have to make it fast, you have to deny its demands, you have to suppress, to repress—they call it *tapas*. That is really twisting the word *tapas* that Patanjali used. I'm not talking about Hatha Yoga, I'm talking about Raja Yoga, and the implications of these words in the whole of Raja Yoga, given by Patanjali.

We are concerned with relating our lives and our way of living with certain truths that were perceived thousands of years ago. We can relate to the truths, not the traditions or structures or codes of conduct.

Tapas is not mortification. No suppression, no repression, no denial—but it is an austerity. And what is that austerity? To live the truth you understand. If you understand the truth about diet, then you do not move an inch away from your understanding about diet. That is *tapas*. If you understand something about sleep, how much sleep is necessary, when to give the body sleep, what kind of bed should be given, then you live that truth. That is *tapas*. What kind of exercises to be given, what clothes to be worn, how to sit the body, how to stand it, how to use speech, how to use sound, how to use the mind, and the movement of thought—once you get acquainted with it, observe it, understand it, then you live the understanding. That is *tapas*.

Why is it called *tapas?* Because we are the products of millions of years of activity. Our bodies, our brains are heavily conditioned, they are programmed through centuries, and therefore the programmed neurochemical system has many habits. Sometimes, though the understanding takes place, the flesh being weak, the thought being rigid, the knowledge being sterile—the body, the mind, the neurochemical system has not the sensitivity to live the understanding. There is rigidity, there is stiffness, and therefore the understanding cannot be lived.

So *tapas* is to educate the body—asanas, pranayama, pratyahara, etc. You educate the body in speech, in ideas, etc., so that it can set itself free of the clutches of conditionings. You cannot destroy conditionings, but you can release yourself from their hold, their domination, their clutches. So *tapas* is required to live the understanding, to live the truth you understood, to educate the body in an alternative way of living—that is called *tapas*.

Austerity is required to live the truth you have perceived. If you do not perceive the truth, there cannot be any *tapas,* because you will be passively repeating certain codes of conduct. *Tapas* requires the alertness and the creativity of your own perception. Purification of your cognition, purification of your neurochemical system, and liberation from the clutches of conditionings—that is the essence of Raja Yoga.

Svādhyāya

Svādhyāya is study. Whatever you want to do, you have to study for it. You have to study books and discuss them with people. If you are doing asanas and pranayama, you will have to study. You will have to go to a teacher to learn asanas, to learn pranayama. In pranayama, you are dealing with the breathing system, which is very delicate. You need someone who has done it before to guide you.

The word *svādhyāya* includes reading, discussing, dialogue, finding a guide to help you do it correctly.

Īśvara Praṇidhāna

The word *īśvara* is translated as "God." I have not seen all the commentaries in French or German because I do not know those languages, but one has come across many commentaries on Indian philosophy and Patanjali Yoga in English. One has looked through those commentaries and one finds that the word *īśvara* has been translated as "God," and to me it seems that "God" does not convey the real sense of *īśvara*.

The word *īśvara* is derived from the root "*īśa*." *Īśate* —"permeates." *Īśate rajate iti īśvarah*. *Īśate* is "to permeate." That which permeates everything is *īśvara*. The word *īśvara* refers to the principle of fundamental Intelligence, the Supreme Intelligence that permeates Life. It is not referring to a god—personal or impersonal, male or female, one or many.

Sankhya refers to it in one way, but Patanjali in Raja Yoga refers to it in a very clear and emphatic way. So the word *īśvara* relates to the all-permeating principle of Supreme Intelligence. In our modern language you can call it the energy of Intelligence that is omnipresent, omnipotent, omniscient, which has an inexhaustible potential of Creativity. The energy of Intelligence, the energy of Creativity permeating Life is *īśvara*. These clarifications seem to be very necessary for the study of Raja Yoga, and they may be necessary if somebody wants to study Vedanta or the Upanishads in India.

Īśvara praṇidhāna. The word *praṇidhāna* is translated as "surrender," and they say if you want to study Raja Yoga, you have to surrender to God. It's a very gross way of translating the word. *Praṇidhāna* would be "to feel" —not to surrender, but to feel the presence of Creativity surrounding you and within you. See, the sages, the rishis who wrote the Vedas, the Upanishads, the Yoga Sutras, they felt it, they had the quality of sensitivity. Where there is sensitivity you get the feel of it. Sensitivity has a quality of perception. Sensitivity perceives, as you perceive through a word, sensitivity perceives through the whole of your being. So we feel the presence of the creative energy around us.

Patanjali says that the feel of the presence of Divinity, of the presence of Creativity, of the presence of Intelligence gets converted into awareness.

Patanjali is referring to the awareness of the presence of Divinity around you. Divinity equal to Intelligence and Creativity. Unqualified Intelligence, unqualified Creativity.

Īśvara praṇidhāna is the last of the niyamas. It is the awareness of the Divinity around you.

CHAPTER SIX

The Yoga of Action

Tapaḥ svādhyāya īśvara-praṇidhānāni kriyāyogaḥ (II.1)

Patanjali codified the sutras that contain or verbalize the truth that was experienced by those who lived before him. Patanjali codified, systematized, and Patanjali Yoga is a science. It is a science of purification of the body and the brain, which is generally called the mind. So obviously the study of the human biological structure and the human psychological structure was done by the ancestors and the forefathers of Patanjali. Being a science of psychophysical purification, it was extremely precise and every word has a particular meaning. We are not free to interpret the words of Patanjali as we are free to interpret the words of Ishavasya Upanishad or other Upanishads. The words of the Vedas and the Upanishads will yield to fresh interpretations as long as the race inhabits the globe, but when it comes to codified sciences like Sankhya, Yoga, Nyaya, Vaishaishika, Purva Mimamsa, and Uttar Mimamsa, or Vedanta, the rishis codified them, and they have accurate and precise meanings for the words, as scientists would have.

So the first thing we note is that the words used by Patanjali have to be understood according to Patanjali. Fortunately, the words of *tapas, svādhyāya,* and *praṇidhāna* have been explained by him, elaborated upon by him in the after-part of that chapter.

It begins with *tapaḥ svādhyāya īśvara-praṇidhānāni kriyāyogaḥ* (II.1), it begins with that, and at the end of the same chapter in the last few sutras the clarification and elaboration is given:

kāya-indriya-siddhir aśuddhi-kṣayāt tapasaḥ (II.43)
svādhyāyād iṣṭa-devatā-saṃprayogaḥ (II.44)
samādhi-siddhir īśvara-praṇidhānāt (II.45)

Tapas

kāya-indriya-siddhir aśuddhi-kṣayāt tapasaḥ (II.43).

Indriya—"sense organs," *śuddhi-karaṇa* —"for purification." For the purification of the sense organs, *tapas* is necessary. The students of yoga have to go through *tapas,* or discipline. Discipline not created by you, but as propounded by the experts who studied the biological structure before Patanjali. So *tapas* is disciplining for the sake of purification. And what are you going to discipline? Your senses, the sensual structure. The eyes, the ears, the nose, the palate, the hands, the feet, the muscular system, the glandular system, the nervous system—all have to be disciplined. Discipline implies, does it not, training? And during training you have to do the same thing, day after day. Training need not become mechanical, repetitive if it is gone through every day or every time with an understanding of the purpose of the discipline.

Tapas is to discipline with the understanding why the discipline is necessary. If the why and how of it are understood, then the process of training, the process of disciplining becomes *tapas*.

So *kāya-indriya-siddhir aśuddhi-kṣayāt tapasaḥ*. For the purification of the senses, *tapas*—the austerity of training, of disciplining—is necessary, it has to be gone through. May I use the term? It is a must.

Now the gross body, the body composed of flesh, blood, bones, tissues, nerves, arteries, muscles, glands—the whole structure marvelously organized into a harmonious whole by nature—has a momentum. Since the first human being that inhabited the globe, these senses have been conditioned. In order to live with nature outside, man has gone through conditioning in his body. The biological structure shares impulses with the rest of the biological world, like the animals, the plants, the minerals, etc. It has impulses built into the system.

The body has these impulses, and their momentum or movement is not created by the race but is a part of cosmic Life; purification implies creating an order, an orderliness and a harmony between the demands of the body. We have to train the body. It has an impulse to sleep, and you have to train the body when to sleep, how much to sleep. There is a demand for food and water, and you have to train the body about the quality, the frequency of intake, and regulate it according to the change of seasons, the change of occupation, the change in the state of the body, the state of mind, and so on. This is training. You have to train the body, teach it and train it.

There is purification through training, purification through education, and purification through sublimation.

Here, purification is to eliminate the imbalances, the tendency toward imbalance, tendency toward excess, tendency toward exaggeration. The real purpose of *tapas,* the real purpose of austerity is to create a harmony in the movement of so many impulses that exist.

Training of the gross body, training of the senses also becomes necessary because we are surrounded by the proliferation of consumer goods, of sensual pleasure, of sensual gratification. You call it a proliferation of goods when it is created by human beings, and when it is natural, you call it a variety.

There is an unaccountable variety in nature of fruits, roots, vegetables, nuts. You have to investigate, explore, and find out which are agreeable to the body and which are not. The disciplining, the austerity comes there. You have to find out which agree with the system and then stick to them, even if your mind is attracted to other kinds of fruits, other kinds of roots and nuts. So the body requires a kind of training. The physical senses require training.

If the *indriyāni*, the senses, are left alone to their impulses and their instincts, they go wild. This morning they want one thing, the next hour they want another thing. They can have contradictory, conflicting movements, and they may ruin your life. They by themselves are not the problem, but the wildness and the chaos that they can create is the problem if they are not channeled. Their movements have to be channeled, they have to be given a purpose, they have to be given a direction—otherwise, they will run amuck like horses. That is *tapas,* or discipline.

Through training, restraint has to be learned. You know, like the reins of a horse, if a horse while cantering or galloping goes wild, you have to pull the reins to control it, regulate it. Not for torturing the horse, but you have to regulate and control in order to create a harmony between your movement and the movement of the horse if you are riding the horse. Before Patanjali, in the Upanishads and the Vedas, the body is compared to a horse. The senses are compared to horses, and the sense of restraint is compared to reins—the intellect is used as a rein and it restrains.

In disciplining, training is implied. In training, restraint is implied. So investigation, exploration, experimentation, training, restraining, and the austerity of sticking to what you have discovered, all this comes under the word *tapas*.

Svādhyāya

Then we come to the term *svādhyāya*.

If one had the freedom to translate or interpret according to one's perception or understanding, one would interpret *svādhyāya* in more than a dozen ways, but we have to stick to what the science of Raja Yoga, what the sutras imply, what Patanjali wants to indicate, and I cannot, you cannot, we cannot impose our meaning upon what Patanjali wants to say. You cannot impose your meaning of words on Sankhya. You can do it with the Bhagavad Gita, which comes after the Upanishads, you can do it with the Upanishads, but not with the six systems of Indian philosophy. It is impossible.

Here, it seems to me, Patanjali interprets *svādhyāya* in two ways. One is the study of the books or scriptures that have gone before him. He says to know about the body, know about the mechanism of mind and thought, know about the brain and cerebral ways of functioning, that knowledge is necessary. In *svādhyāya* he is referring to knowledge very explicitly. You have to study what is the body, how does it work, what is thought, what is the brain, what are their interactions and interrelations. *Svādhyāya* is studying the books about human life written before the time of Patanjali—that is one aspect of *svādhyāya*; the other is study through observation.

For observing how the mind moves, for observing how the instincts and impulses move, first you have to study. You have to study for the sake of knowledge and then study through observation. Your observation converts knowing into understanding. Because in yoga you are dealing with a living organism, which is conditioned by nature, by so many energies, knowledge is necessary about the human body and brain as much as knowledge is necessary about a motorcar or a computer. You cannot decode the language of a computer unless you have studied it. So when I have to decode so many things in my mind and brain, knowledge is a necessity. That is what Patanjali's Yoga Sutras have to say.

Patanjali says refer to the books, study the books of the seers who have gone before us. *Sūri* is a word used for "wise man," *sūri* is the word used for "a seer." *Purva* is "those who have gone before." After having studied the books, observe it in your own life, because knowledge does not become understanding unless and until it is verified by your personal observations. You have to verify what has been known through observations, because through observations you have contact with the fact. With study, you had knowledge of the fact, not contact. The contact was indirect, through words—words coined, formulated, organized by others—but through observation you have direct, immediate, intimate contact with the fact and therefore a communion with the fact. Observation results in communion with the fact, knowledge prepares the background, knowledge gives information about the fact, so *svādhyāya* is both study and observation.

A student of yoga will have to spend some part of his day, some time of the day practicing *tapas,* that is to say, the yamas, the niyamas, the asanas, pranayama. He has to spend some of his time in this and some of his time in study and observation—*kriyāyoga.*

So *kriyāyoga* is the yoga of activity and action both; *kriyāyoga* includes *tapas* and *svādhyāya.*

Svādhyāya—study—purifies the brain. If there was ignorance, the ignorance is dispelled; if there was wrong information, it gets rectified and corrected; if there was lack of information or ignorance, it gets eliminated.

You can get the information through the words of those who have gone before us, those who have experimented themselves, those who have done the *sādhana.*

Therefore the brain gets purified. There is an elimination of imbalances, elimination of incorrect information and ignorance. And through illumination there is contact with the words of those who lived those words. Purification through *svādhyāya. Svādhyāya*—the study part—cleanses the intellect of all ignorance, of all imbalances, of all impurities. After having cleansed the brain through study, the observation purifies.

Now what is the difference between clarity and purification? When clarity crystallizes as a dimension, it becomes the substance of your being. Then there is no scope, there is no possibility of ignorance, incorrectness, or imbalances coming back to the brain, then you can call it purity. If you do not observe the facts, you might forget what is studied and forgetfulness may again create the darkness of ignorance. If you have only studied and not observed, not seen the facts for yourself, then what is studied can be forgotten. But when what is seen, perceived, and communed with becomes the substance of your life, the clarity that was arrived at through intellectual study, through verbal study gets purified through observations and direct intimate contact and communion with Reality. There is then no possibility of forgetting. It is no more a part of your memory—it has become the substance of your being. You have observed it, you have seen it. Once you have seen the light, you never confuse it with darkness. Once clarity is arrived at, not only through words but through personal perception and observations, then there is the dimension of purity, which becomes the substance of your being—incorruptible, undamageable, inaccessible to confusion.

Īśvara Praṇidhāna

Tapas, svādhyāya, and last we come to *īśvara praṇidhāna.* Sankhya does not use the term *īśvara* and Patanjali uses the term *īśvara praṇidhāna. Tapaḥ svādhyāya īśvara-praṇidhānāni kriyāyogaḥ* (II.1). He uses the word *īśvara,* but *īśvara* does not refer to a personal god. The term *īśvara* used by Patanjali does not refer to any man-made god, any god which is a creation of human thought or human hand. Perhaps no temples or mosques or churches or organized religions existed when he lived. Then why does he use the term *īśvara?* The Yoga Sutras were codified in 553 B.C. What was then the relevance of using the term *īśvara?* This point has to be very clearly understood to discriminate between paganism and what Patanjali had to say.

Do you know what paganism is? They deify everything. The tree is a god, the bird is a god, the river is a god or goddess, the mountain is a god. Among tribal people you still get these ideas, and if you exclude Africa, the greatest number of tribals live in India.

So in paganism everything is a god or goddess, and that god or goddess has a mind, and that god or goddess can get angry. It can become favorable or unfavorable to you, it can do damage to you if it gets angry and it can give rewards if it is pleased. You know the god/goddess getting pleased or angry or destroying—that is paganism. Patanjali was not a pagan. He is not referring to particular gods and goddesses, he has no concept of that, he is referring purely, simply to the word *īśvara* as a principle that permeates life. The whole world is permeated by that principle. He does not call it Intelligence, he does not give it a name. He does not refer to the word *god*, he does not refer to the word *divine*, he just says, "that which permeates everything." To refer to it, there must be a code language, code words.

Īśvara praṇidhāna —the attitude of surrender, the attitude of recognizing the all-pervasiveness or all-permeatingness. When you recognize it intellectually and you accept it psychologically, it becomes surrender. Surrender is nothing more. Surrender is not giving up your efforts, surrender is not becoming a slave to it. *Praṇidhāna*—I'm translating it as "surrender" because I don't find a better word.

Recognize that there is a principle that transcends matter and energy, which transcends all the structures—which is innate in them and yet transcendent. There is a principle permeating everything, due to which there is order in the world, due to which there is harmony in the world, due to which the movement of life becomes possible.

Patanjali says that while making effort, while training, while studying, become aware that there is a principle permeating everything. Toward It, have an attitude of surrender—otherwise you might mistake yourself as the master of your body and master of the cosmos or the universe. You are in a limited form and all your actions are limited. You have to work in a conditioned, limited structure, so whatever you do has limitation. But there is an unlimited, all-pervading principle that is omniscient, omnipresent, omnipotent—these three beautiful terms explain everything that is indicated by the word *īśvara*. There is no other meaning to the word *īśvara* as far as Patanjali is concerned.

Now if one recognizes the existence and the functioning of the principle that transcends the human body, the human brain, and all that is seen around us, if there is a principle innate and yet transcendent, permeating the whole and operating in and through everything, what does this recognition do to us? Will it not evoke an attitude of surrender in us?

Life is a dance of the nameable and the unnameable, of temporary imbalances and eternal equipoise, or equanimity, of emergence and dissolution. Life is a dance of all that. If we recognize *īśvara,* the presence of the all-permeating principle, then we understand the dance of Life, the cosmic dance of Life.

If I have recognized the other and realized the nature of the dance, what is this realization going to do to the quality of my life? I have to function through the center of the "Me," the "I," the monitor of the psychophysical structure, the monitor of the biological structure. We have to function from the center, from the center of the "Me," the ego, which is only a conceptual center, which is only an ideational center. We should never mistake it for the reality of our essence. That is not the essence of our being. So though we function from it, there is no self-centeredness. Though we function from it, we do not get attached to the ego. We function from it because that is a necessity. Just as we do not drop our bodies but function through them, though they are limited and Life is unlimited and infinite.

As we function through the limitations of the body, which is going to die one day, we function through the center of the "Me," but that center does not become a problem, we do not become addicted to it because we are aware of the *īśvara*. All that you do, what you think is really dedicated to the *īśvara*. It is an offering to the *īśvara*—the all-permeating, pervasive principle.

How do you express *praṇidhāna?* To me, an elegant, magnificent, majestic humility is the content of surrender—*praṇidhāna*. Ego does not know humility. Ego is assertive, aggressive, acquisitive, competitive.

So reminding yourself of the all-permeating, pervading principle of Life, the dynamism of Life, the petty little center does not become all-important. You use it, you handle it, you function through it, but you do not get attached to it, you do not become dependent on it. You use it as you use the body, and when the movement is not necessary, you are in *īśvara praṇidhāna*.

Refinement and purification of the whole cerebral and neurochemical system through study and observation, purification of the gross body through training, teaching, restraining is necessary. The student of yoga spends his day in *tapaḥ svādhyāya īśvara-praṇidhānāni kriyāyogaḥ*. If you do the first two and there is no awareness of the *īśvara,* no awareness of the presence of the *īśvara* around you and within you, then you can become very arrogant, you can become very self-centered, isolatory, etc.

Patanjali Yoga has a kind of devotion and dedication to *īśvara,* which I call the Supreme Intelligence.

CHAPTER SEVEN

The Kleshas

Avidyā-asmitā-rāga-dveṣa-abhiniveśāḥ kleśāḥ (II.3)

Question: What are the fivefold kleshas, and what can one do to get free of them in daily living?

The words in the question are of great significance, and we should look at those words before we proceed to find out what the fivefold kleshas are and what can be done about them.

The questioner says in the second part of the question: "What can we do to get free of the kleshas in our daily life?" There is no other life except what you call "the daily life." The day, the today, the now, the here—what you call this moment is the only reality for you and me. To meet it, to live through it. Life is relationship and the movement of relationship is living. To live is to be related. To be related to and interact with human beings, nonhuman beings, nature at large constitutes what you call life.

So let us amend the question: "What can be done to be free of the kleshas in life, in the midst of the movement of relationship?" Not as an abstract theory, not academically, but practically, in every moment, in every relationship.

Kleśa

If that is clear, let us look at the word *kleśa*. The questioner has used the phrase five kleshas.

What is *kleśa?* How do you translate that into English? Do you translate it as pain, as hurt, or as suffering? For the English words "pain" and "hurt," there is a Sanskrit word *dukham. Dukham* and *sukham. Sukham* is defined as "agreeable sensation." "Disagreeable sensation" is *dukham.*

So *kleśa* and *dukham,* they are two different things. We cannot avoid *dukham.* Pain, hurt cannot be avoided, as long as we are living. Climatic changes, changes of surroundings, congenital sickness in the body, hereditary sickness, or distortions of the body can cause pain. If you come across something that causes a disagreeable sensation, the body has to go through the event of pain. That pain is a psychophysical event, and it is bound to take place while we are living, because we are not the creators or controllers of climate or surroundings, etc.

In the same way, you can use the word "hurt" also as a synonym for *dukham* on the physical level. Biological pain is equal to *dukham.* On the psychological level the sensitivity can be hurt, as the foot gets hurt if pricked by a thorn. You can call it pain or you can call it hurt. If the sensitivity is refined, then if one has to witness or one has to go through relationships where people behave crudely, unaesthetically, where there is inaccuracy of behavior, where there is roughness, harshness, lack of precision, then the aesthetically keen sensitivity, the refined sensitivity experiences an acute hurt. It is not physical. Nobody has touched your body but inside the sensitivity gets hurt; that also is *dukham.*

On the psychophysical level, it seems to me that *dukham,* or pain or hurt, cannot be avoided. It takes place as an event. But this is not called *kleśa.*

I'm trying, with your cooperation, to look at the meaning of the word *kleśa.* The word *kleśa* could be translated into English by the word "suffering." When the pain or hurt that took place in a fraction of a moment is given continuity by thought, when there is identification with it, when there is identification with the event that took place, and you say, "I was hurt," "I was insulted," "I was humiliated," then there is suffering. The event took place objectively—you cannot deny it, you cannot avoid it. Ramana Maharshi, Shri Ramakrishna, Shri Krishnamurti, they could not avoid the disease of cancer in their bodies, and they must have gone through tremendous pain—pain to the body. Pain is one thing, and it takes place as an event; suffering is inflicted by thought, which gives it continuity. Identification gives continuity.

So *kleśa* is suffering, misery with the help of imagination due to fear, due to identification. Out of the physical pain and hurt we create suffering—psychological suffering. *Kleśa* is psychological suffering. Please let us not translate *kleśa* by the words "pain" or "hurt," otherwise it will be an inaccurate translation.

If the meaning of these two words is sufficiently clear, let us proceed to the *pañca kleśāḥ*. *Pañca* means "five." You can say fivefold or five.

What are the five kleshas according to Patanjali? *Avidyā-asmitā-rāga-dveṣa-abhiniveśāḥ kleśāḥ* (II.3).

Patanjali defines, enumerates, explains the fivefold suffering which human beings go through and which, according to him, is not warranted. That suffering can be avoided, that suffering can be transcended. You can put an end to that suffering. The *pañca kleśāḥ* can be ended. Religion ends the psychological suffering, but not the physical pain and hurt. That does not seem possible except for persons who have studied Hatha Yoga and specialized in Hatha Yoga, where they can add longevity to the body and they can avoid physical sicknesses, diseases. If you specialize in Hatha Yoga, it is possible, to a very great extent, to avoid even physical pain and sicknesses.

Patanjali Yoga is Raja Yoga. Though the Ashtanga Yoga of Hatha Yoga is included in Raja Yoga, it is only a very small part. The Ashtanga Yoga of yamas, niyamas, asanas, pranayama, etc., is only a part of Raja Yoga, not the essence, as it is in Hatha Yoga.

Avidyā

Vidyā—"self-knowledge." I'm talking about the Sanskrit language of the period of the Vedas, the Upanishads and the six systems of Indian philosophy—Sankhya, Yoga, etc. I'm talking of the Sanskrit language and its meaning of that period. If you go today to India and ask somebody what is *vidyā*, they will say, "knowledge." That was not the implication for Patanjali.

It has been written that *vidyā* means "*adhyātma*." What is *adhyātma*? Understanding yourself, knowing what you are. *Avidyā* is ignorance about one's own nature, ignorance about one's existential essence, about one's own being. Not ignorance about chemistry, physics, etc.—that is not the meaning or the connotation of the term *avidyā*. Here in Patanjali's Yoga Sutras or in Ishavasya Upanishad, the word *avidyā* refers to ignorance about one's own nature, one's own essence. If there is ignorance about the essence of one's being, then one would identify and equate one's wholeness with things that are smaller, that are compartmental, that are fragmentary. If I do not understand what Life is, what the Is-ness of Life is, what the Suchness of Life is, then I identify with things that are smaller.

Suchness is the term used by the Buddhists. *Is-ness* is the word used by the Vedantins. *Satta* or "to-be-ness" is the expression your friend Vimala generally uses for communicating the essence.

If the to-be-ness which is here, functioning, operating, is not understood properly, is not perceived, if you do not get acquainted with the inner substance of your being, the content of being, the mechanism of the to-be-ness, then it is quite possible that you think this body is you—"I am the body and the body is Me." There can be wrong identification and when the body becomes sick you say, "I am sick" or if the body is dying you say, "I am dying." It is a wrong equation, it is a wrong identification. Most often it happens that there is wrong equation and wrong identification. Some people do not equate the biological structure with the essence of their being, they equate their knowledge, their thoughts with the essence of their being, they equate their views, their memory with the essence of their being. So they say, "I am hurt" or "This is my possession" or "This is my experience—sensual, extrasensory, transcendental." They go on identifying with the experiences, the pieces of knowledge, and they think that the to-be-ness, the Is-ness is equal to memory, knowledge, experience, values, etc., and then suffering begins.

When there is not the identification with the body and when there is freedom of awareness, then the essence of life is not only the physical structure, its movements, its birth, its decay, its death, then the essence of life is something additional, something qualitatively different. Then the identification does not take place, therefore there is no *kleśa,* there is no suffering.

It is only when the pain enters the mind, that is to say, when there is the identification, and you say, "I am suffering," not "There is pain in the body" but "I am in pain," that the *kleśā* begins.

Avidyā is ignorance about the essence of one's being. In one's being there is also this psychophysical body. Like the crust of bread, like the skin of fruit, it is necessary. Without the body, the essence, the energy of Intelligence, the creativity—whatever you call it—cannot manifest itself. The very manifestation requires the form, the very expression requires the form, so the form also is part of that, but it is like the skin of the fruit. If you identify with the sensation of the self, of the "Me," which is finer than the gross body and give continuity to the hurt that has taken place, then there is suffering. It was the sensitivity that was hurt, it was a sense of self-respect that was hurt, it was an image about yourself that was disturbed. It does happen and in relationships such moments cannot be avoided, but then the thought gives continuity—this happened to me, she did it to me, he did it to me. That suffering is the result of thought conferring continuity, that is to say, the domination of the idea of psychological time. Thought is time really speaking, so thought gives continuity and pain becomes suffering.

Patanjali says, when this basic ignorance about the essence of one's being is eliminated and there is *vidyā,* when there is self-knowing, self-understanding, when there is the discovery of the essence of one's being, then the *kleśa* called *avidyā,* the *kleśa* caused by *avidyā* gets eliminated, it gets ended once and for all.

Asmitā

The next is *asmitā.* The word *asmitā* is translated generally by most of the commentators—Indian and non-Indian—as "egoism." Some call it egoism, some call it egotism. To look upon the wholeness of your life as only the movement of the ego, the self, the "Me" is *asmitā.*

The body is an individual body, but the movement of thought, the movement of knowledge, experience, inheritance inside the body, the movement of programming and conditioning, the impression of those conditionings in the body, has a particularity—not an individuality—of expression. Like a particular model of car from a factory of cars, there is a particular expression of collectively standardized, organized, sanctioned neurochemical ways of behavior, which you call mental behavior. The mental movement is going to be there. Thought structure or the programmed and conditioned psychophysical structure is there, you cannot escape from it and you have to use the words *I* and *me.* But please see that it has only ideational reality, not a factual content. The body has a factual content—flesh and blood and bones—but inside the conditionings and programmings have a vibrational existence permeating the whole body.

The "I," the ego has only a particularity of expression, not an individuality of an entity. There is no entity within the body. We imagine that there must be an ego, a self, a *jīva,* a soul, and so on. We transfer that, or rather we extend that idea from the biological, the physical to the psychological, but there is only a collectively produced cerebral and neurochemical way of behavior—mechanistic, repetitive, automatic movements and reactions to the pattern of conditioning.

Sometimes we identify the wholeness of Life with this idea, with the concept of the "Me." This is like the point in geometry, if you want to define the point you can't, you may say it has no length, no breadth, but put a point on the paper and you may say it has both. The arithmetical numbers—1, 2, 3 up to 99—they are our creations, and we say 2 + 3 = 5, this is our counting, this is our measurement, this is our scale. There are no numbers in Reality, but these are our measures. In the same way, the ego has the same kind of reality as the arithmetical numbers have, they have the same kind of reality as your words and languages have. The word is not the thing—it only points to the existence of something, it is a pointer.

Asmitā is identification with the ideational structure. *Avidyā* is confusing the essence of being with something that it is not, and *asmitā* is identifying the whole knowledge with the essence of your being. There is a movement of knowledge without a knower inside, there is a movement of experiencing without an experiencer. That is the only way of going through the events. You go through an event—the stimulus applied inside creates an impulse, awakening memory, memory interprets the event—and then you say, "It is my experience." Light was perceived and then you say, "I saw the light." "Ah, that was an occult experience." Perception of light, perception of sound may be a fact, may be just an event, but the event gets converted into an experience when you refer it back to memory and identify it, compare it, evaluate it, and give it a name.

There may be the movement of experiencing without the experiencer, and the movement of knowledge and the playback or reaction of the conditionings without the entity inside, which perhaps does not exist at all.

Asmitā is identification with the conceptual structure, and it becomes the cause of suffering. How does it become the cause of suffering? The biological body, the physical structure, it has to be preserved, so you have to have food, clothing, shelter. You have to take care of its health, etc., there is an urge to preserve it, an urge to defend it against the odds of life, to protect it, to see it continue unobstructed, there is an urge incorporated into the biological structure, a sense of security, a sense of preservation. Now that gets extended and we naively believe that the "I" has to be protected, as the body has to be protected. As the body has to have a house, the "I" must have the house of thought to live in, the house of knowledge to live in. It must have the protection of defense mechanisms, it must have the protection of a code of conduct, it must be given all this. As there are methods and techniques of preservation of the physical body we keep this, and we extend the physical fear to the psychological level. We extend the idea of security to the psychological level, and that is how suffering is inflicted by ourselves on ourselves.

Rāga–dveṣa

After a few aphorisms, Patanjali defines *rāga* and *dveṣa* both:

sukhānuśayī rāgaḥ (II.7)

duḥkhānuśayī dveśaḥ (II.8)

The desire for repetition of pleasure results in attachment. *Rāga* is "attachment" in English, so he calls *rāga* or attachment a source of suffering, a cause of suffering, or even an expression of suffering. *Rāga* is suffering. Wrong identification leads to suffering. There is nothing wrong with pleasure. None of the Vedas, the Upanishads, or the six systems of Indian philosophy have ever said that you should avoid pleasure, that you should invite pain, that you should mortify the body and torture it. They have not said it because they are worshippers of Life and they are lovers of Life.

Sukhānuśayī rāgaḥ. There is nothing wrong with pleasure. We have beautiful senses in the human body. Your eyes see colors, beautiful shapes and you have pleasure, maybe for a fraction of a second. If you want the pleasure to continue, then you are creating suffering, but by itself the contact of sight with the various shapes, sizes, colors is beautiful. You have flowers with scents—rose, lotus—and they do something to your whole body when you get that fragrance. It is a momentary pleasure. It is only when you want that pleasure to be repeated, and for the repetition of the pleasure you want to capture the object or the individual that has caused the pleasure and you want to own it, possess it, cling to it, dominate it, exploit it, him, or her, that there is suffering.

Rāga—the desire to repeat the pleasure results in attachment, and attachment is another source of *kleśa,* or suffering.

Rāga and *dveṣa* are two sides of a coin. On one side is what you call *rāga* and on the other side of the coin is *dveṣa. Dveṣa* is "aversion." The desire to run away, to avoid. "Repulsion" would be a stronger term. Disinclination to have any contact, dislike, when a dislike becomes permanent, when it gets crystallized, you call it aversion—it may be momentary, transitory, temporary. Today you dislike it, after a month you like it. So likes and dislikes are floating. They may change but once the like crystallizes, it becomes infatuation, obsession, and once the dislike crystallizes, it can become aversion and, if it gets still stronger, repulsion.

Duḥkhānuśayī dveśaḥ (II.8)—Patanjali describes it as the desire to manipulate life in such a way that there will not be any suffering. Trying to run away from pain and hurt. Being afraid of pain and hurt, you create dislike, aversion, repulsion, hatred. *Dveṣa* could be translated as "hatred" also.

Attachment does not allow you to live in freedom, because once you get attached to objects you form a habit pattern. When you get attached to individuals and you feel you can't live without them, or you make yourself indispensable to other people, then the suffering begins.

When there is a reluctance to see that *dukham*—pain—cannot be avoided, when there is a reluctance to see this fact, then there is *kleśa.* Buddha must have seen this deep-rooted tendency in human beings to ignore *dukham* as part of life; that is why he says "*Sarvam dukham, sarvam śānikam.*"

There is pain in life, you can't avoid it, so do not run away from it. But that does not mean that you go and invite pain and become a sadist, it does not mean morbid habits of torturing the body, not that thing, but that pleasure and pain both are unavoidable. One need not be afraid of pleasure, that it will excite, and so run away from it. One need not be afraid of pain, that it will create a permanent imbalance, and so run away from it. When you recognize pleasure and pain—*sukham* and *dukham*—as parts of life, then there is no *kleśa.*

You have asked me about the *pañca kleśāḥ,* and the last is *abhiniveśa.*

Abhiniveśa

Let me see how to approach this *abhiniveśa.* Aggressive inclination to cling to the body, aggressive inclination, let me say even an ambition, to cling to the body. I'm studying with you, looking at what Patanjali said. When there is an aggressive desire, not only inclination, not even impulse, but a desire to cling to the body, the physical body, then there is fear of dying and death.

Obsession with the body, to protect it at any cost, at every cost, to preserve it at any cost and every cost, one is afraid to live, one is afraid of life. Supposing I do this, it might hurt my body, supposing I do that, it might hurt my mind.

Abhiniveśa is a kind of suffering which is the result of this obsession with the body, not only identification but you are infatuated, obsessed with the body. The body becomes the center of all your attention, a vested interest is there in the preservation and the continuity of the body. So there is no openness, no receptivity to open out in relationship, to open out to life. There is always the overprotectiveness and you isolate yourself.

Abhiniveśa isolates. *Abhiniveśa* does not allow you to mix with people, to be with them, it is an inhibition in the movement of relationships. You are always on your guard. You have an image of yourself that has to be protected. Your body has to be protected, its likes and dislikes have to be protected. So there is a kind of inhibition, an overprotective impulse that always keeps you in a shell, as it were, it doesn't allow you to open up your doors and windows to life. You weave around yourself a nest of your knowledge, your inheritance, your ideologies, etc., and you keep yourself protected. You can't receive anything new. If a new communication, if something fresh comes to you that is different from the nest that you had built up, straw by straw, gathering pieces of knowledge, you are afraid that it will be destroyed, so you stick to the old, you cling to the old. *Abhiniveśa* does not allow you to live creatively, does not allow you to die creatively—to meet death as the culmination of the act of living. It does not allow you, because it fills you with a nameless fear, with a faceless fear. Not fear of anything particular but fear of everything.

The second part of the question is, "What do you do to get free of these kleshas in living?"

I wonder if you have faith in your perception, if you trust your psychological perception, as you trust your physical perception? You see a snake and there is an instantaneous response of the whole being. Perception and the response of the whole being—there is no time lag in between, because you trust your perception of a physical fact. Unfortunately, the human race has not cultivated the sensitivity through education to respond to the perception of a psychological fact without a time lag. We respond to a physical fact without a time lag at all, and it is not a mechanical response. In the presence of danger the intelligence of the person works, the organic intelligence immediately responds.

Perception of a psychological fact has to take place through the sight of sensitivity—not these physical eyes, but the other eyes. Sensitivity is a perception. You feel it, you perceive it, but then there is a time lag. We feel, "Yes, I have seen it. Now tell me what to do about it." Do you see the difference? It is not a question of you and me, it is not a question of individuals. We—you and I—represent the whole human race. After having inhabited the globe for so many centuries, there is so much to learn and the human race is so slow to learn. It has not educated itself. Now, however, education in the perception of psychological facts has begun. The emergence of psychology, parapsychology as a science is a recent phenomenon of the last hundred years or so.

Now we are learning to objectify inner movements, to verbalize about them, to look at them. Verbalization of the psychological fact and fearless perception of the fact—these two things have taken place in the global life of the human race. But the third step is left, there is a missing link. The response does not come spontaneously from the wholeness of being, because we have been nourished on knowledge, we have been nourished on words—the nutrition has been of words and theories and ideas and concepts. First you acquire knowledge, then society provides you with the incentives—if you are virtuous you go to heaven, if you commit sins you go to hell. Rewards, punishments are offered in religion, in ethics, in politics, in economics. First know, then provide incentives, then codes of conduct.

If there is a time lag between knowing and living, it is because knowledge comes in between. The chain of incentives, the code of conduct, the instructions inhibit the sensitivity. The sensitivity does not respond immediately. And now due to the study of yoga or meditation as a way of living, the human race sees the urgency of activating the sensitivity, so that there is no time lag between the perception of psychological fact and the response from the whole being.

We are in the transitional period. Two important steps have been taken by the human race. The third remains to be taken, and I think the interest in yoga, balanced nutrition, Tai Chi, holistic medicine, experiments in alternative ways of living, alternative culture—all these things that are taking place all over the world, is a global wave in the human consciousness to eliminate this time lag between perception and response.

I'm sharing this with you so that you do not carry any guilt consciousness about yourself that "I cannot respond, I understand, there is verbal knowledge, and yet the change does not take place." One could hold oneself guilty and suffer unnecessarily. It is not an individual failure, it is a missing link in the psychic growth of the human race of which you and I are parts, and now we want to correct it. So without any sense of frustration, guilt consciousness, depression, we should be able to look at the facts as they are.

I have, with the help of words, investigated what the kleshas are. I have verbally understood what the kleshas are. Now let me observe in daily life how this suffering works, how the kleshas operate. Let me watch them in myself. The factual encounter will give the understanding. Now it is only an idea, it remains only a word. However clear, logical, sane, and flawless the exposition might be, still it is only a description and the description is not the described.

Let me see the suffering. Let me feel the pain, the agony, the sorrow of it. Unless you see the nature of bondage, unless you see the heaviness, the darkness of bondage, the urge for liberation does not have vitality, it does not have that passion to break through. It remains only a pious wish and therefore has not got any momentum. Words don't have any momentum.

So the third step would be to watch and have a personal encounter with these five kleshas operating within one's life. And that encounter hurts the sensitivity, it churns your whole being, because the sensitivity, the intelligence does not like to remain a prisoner of all this suffering. The encounter causes a deep sorrow, the observation, the perception of suffering created by *avidyā, asmitā,* etc., causes a deep sorrow, the whole being becomes a flame of sorrow, the kleshas become unbearable. It is the sacred agony of sorrow, the sharpness of sorrow cutting you, as it were. And mind you, friends, these are not mere words, this is Vimala's life, she has gone through it, otherwise she would not have the courage to sit here and talk to you.

Now the ego, the idea of the ego, is torn down to pieces, is shattered, the images that one had about oneself get broken down to pieces, and you see all that is within you and around you. You may call it the dark night of the soul, if you like. That is the language used by the Sufis and the Bhakti Yoga people—the yoga of devotion in India.

If one fearlessly sticks out the sorrow caused by the personal encounter of the operation of the kleshas within one, then the dark night ends with the dawn of a new perspective on life. One does not want to use any poetic language, but life is poetry.

Till this happens, when I notice the suffering in me, when I notice the attachment in me or the aversion, repulsion, hatred in me in my so-called daily living, what do I do? That is the last part of the question. I don't do anything. Please do see this, I don't do anything. I don't go in for therapy, I don't go in for a method or a technique to get rid of it, for whatever is done is going to create a new network of suffering—pleasant in the beginning, painful later on, and you are back in the trap.

It is very important to realize that the "I" cannot do anything to get rid of the kleshas, because the kleshas are a creation of the "I" or the "Me," the self, the ego. To be with the kleshas, to observe, "This is attachment, this is repulsion, this is causing the bitterness, this is giving a smile or grin to my face." Be with it, be with the "I," or rather don't try to run away from it, from your own intelligence. Just be with it, you have seen what it is, you would like to get it eliminated, uprooted, removed completely. That is enough. You have seen, you have understood, now let the dynamism concealed in the perception, let the dynamics contained in understanding operate upon you. As a hangover of the old habit it may come back, let it come back without feeling guilty, without getting depressed, without having self-pity or a sense of frustration. In a very simple, humble way be with what is—maybe it is *rāga, dveṣa, asmitā.* No condemnation, no criticism, no desire to touch it or change it. Just be with it because what you could do, you have done. You got first the verbal information, you got that information by reading, by attending talks, by participating in discussions. You have observed and watched. Whatever you could do, you have done honestly. Now the investigation, the inquiry has to stop, because it has served its purpose, it cannot go any further—every effort by the "I" will create one more complication.

After knowledge and observation, the sacred moment comes to remain effortlessly in the presence of the fact, not ignoring it, not touching it. That is *tapas.* You are being with the fact, with all the perception and understanding contained in you. No eagerness, no impatience, no comparison—"Why hasn't it changed me? Why didn't it happen to me?" Nothing of that, just "I have done what I want to, now I am there, all alert, all attentive but effortless."

The effortlessness of the "I," the "Me," the ego, the unconditional relaxation of the ego would be the greatest contribution, and freedom would be the perfume of that relaxation, of that effortlessness.

CHAPTER EIGHT

Dharana and Dhyana

Before we proceed, I would like to clarify one point. Since the beginning of this camp, Vimala has been trying to share with you her understanding of Patanjali Yoga, of Raja Yoga. She is not singing her song. She will sing her own song in the next camp, but in this camp one is trying one's level best to put into words what one has understood as Patanjali Yoga, what Patanjali must have meant in his aphorisms, the meaning of the Sanskrit words, what they imply literally. I do not bring in the points here whether I agree or disagree with Patanjali. Let us look at him, let us listen to him, and let us understand what he says for students and teachers of yoga. This clarification is necessary, as we shall proceed with a special reference to your questions about *dhāraṇā* and *dhyāna* according to Patanjali.

Question: What is the role of *dhāraṇā* and *dhyāna*? What is the relationship between *dhāraṇā* and *dhyāna* according to Patanjali?

A close scrutiny of Patanjali's words and aphorisms, a scientific, nonauthoritarian study of Patanjali's Sutras, seems to be vitally necessary and we are trying to do it very briefly because we cannot study the whole of Patanjali Yoga in one week. There is the Sadhana Path, the Siddhi Path, the Samadhi Path—so many different chapters—but we are looking at it briefly in a nonsectarian, nondogmatic way. It seems to be a very precise science given to us by *muni* Patanjali.

Let us begin by understanding the role of conditioning in the development of human culture and civilization. In order to understand *dhāraṇā* we have to understand the role of conditioning in our lives, because *dhāraṇā* is the method of concentration in which you are conditioning what you call your mind or what is generally called the thought structure—the psychological structure, that vibrational stuff in the body.

Conditioning can be done or has been done in many ways. We condition the matter around us—the trees, the plants, the earth, the rivers. When we come to the animal world and the world of birds, the conditioning is in the form of training. You make the animals or birds repeat certain movements. You must have heard of Pavlov and his behavioral psychology. You make someone repeat a pattern of behavior—that is what you do with animals when you claim you are taming them.

Training is one way of conditioning. You condition the gross matter, you condition the plant world and you condition the animal kingdom through this process of repetitive, mechanical movement. It does not help the animal or bird to understand why the movement is to be done. Training is one form of conditioning where you do not expect the trainee to use his own initiative or freedom. You just expect the animal or bird to be a passive recipient of what you are doing.

The second aspect of conditioning is education. You educate the child to repeat certain movements. You teach the child how to eat with knife and fork, how to chew, all this is done methodically. Methods and systems are necessary while you are educating children.

What is the difference between the repetition that animals go through and the repetition that human beings go through?

There is a beautiful word in Sanskrit to describe this process of learning through repetition during the educational period. It is called *abhyāsa*. You also come across the aphorism in Patanjali's Yoga Sutras: *abhyāsa vairāgya-ābhyāṃ tan-nirodhaḥ* (I.12).

Here you are expecting the child to learn by repeating. As he grows, he has to repeat words to learn pronunciation, to learn grammar. He has to repeat the rules and regulations and learn certain things by memory. You expect the child to go through this repetition while understanding why it has to be done. You don't want the child to be only a passive animal, you want him to learn. You are helping, through education, which is a process of conditioning. But at the same time you try to stimulate the intelligence of the child, you want the child to understand very clearly why certain kinds of things are to be done.

The child is going to condition his own body, speech, and even his thinking process with your help. So education is helping the child to discipline himself. Education is helping the child to condition himself. If you do not help the child to understand, then it is not education. Here you are stimulating the urge to learn, you are stimulating the taste for learning, the love of learning and of understanding. The process of conditioning is used here for awakening the love of learning and the love of discipline together with the understanding as to why the discipline has to be gone through. So it is not entirely mechanical. It is not entirely repetitive, the repetition has a new element. Please do see the difference between training and education—the two forms of conditioning.

There is a third aspect of conditioning where methods and systems are necessary, where you convert the gross matter into refined and sophisticated matter. You make the matter go through a process of conditioning, and you provoke the latent powers contained and concealed in that matter. We have seen training, we have seen education. Now we are coming to something much deeper.

For example, when you make your body go through the asanas combined with the process of pranayama, you are refining the muscular, the glandular, the nervous system, so that the latent powers contained in the body begin to manifest and get activated.

For example, when you study pranayama there are certain techniques and methods. like learning to retain the breath for longer periods of time. You go on increasing the duration of the *antara kumbhaka,* and thus you can develop the latent powers in the body.

For example, if you learn Tantra Yoga—*dakṣinā* and *vāma,* or the right and the left part of Tantra, as they call it—it is concerned with stimulating the energies contained in significant parts of your body, which they call the chakras. The scientists of Tantra Yoga discovered seven very critical junctures, junctions where different nerves—sensory and motor—meet. These meeting points, which they call chakras, each have a specific power. They talk about the *sahasrāra cakra*—the thousand-petal lotus at the crown of the head. They talk of a *cakra* between the eyebrows, in the heart, in the throat, in the navel point, in the *mūlādhāra,* etc. They are very important, significant points where certain nerves meet, connected with glands. So Tantra Yoga is conditioning those energy channels and those points of nerves—sensory, motor. You condition them so that the latent powers contained in those channels and those points begin to manifest themselves. If you tear the human body, you won't find any chakras in your anatomy. These seven points were developed into seventy points by Hatha Yoga. You will find mention of it in Hatha Yoga Pradipika, and the scientists in their study of acupuncture and acupressure, they have gone into seven hundred different points of the body. You can touch them and awaken the energies for bringing back your health. That is to say that, like blood circulation, there are certain healing energies in the body, if they get blocked somewhere, if their flow gets blocked, then you become ill or sick. So the Chinese went up to seven hundred points. Hatha Yoga talks about seventy points, Tantra Yoga talks about seven points in the body. You condition the matter in order to bring out the latent powers. So this is the third aspect of conditioning that requires a method, that requires a system.

One could go on elaborating upon the variety of the conditioning processes and all the nuances and shades of this human culture. Conditioning is the content of human culture. It is not always for limiting, it is not always for crushing the original. It is helping the original, sophisticating, refining the original, and awakening and provoking the manifestation of the latent energies within. The wealth of human culture, if understood properly and handled properly, can be an asset, but if you do not handle it properly, then even an asset can become a bondage, can become a limitation.

Let us refer to one more approach to this process of conditioning which is *dhāraṇā*.

When you study *dhāraṇā,* it is the method of concentration where you are conditioning what you call your mind or what I generally call the thought structure, the psychological structure—that vibrational stuff inside the body. You are conditioning that stuff which was diffused, running out of the body or even inside the body in different directions to different ideas, to different words, running out to different objects outside the body, and getting diffused. You are conditioning that stuff to come back from the diffused state to a collected, composed, concentrated state. Concentrating the diffused energy is concentration—please do see the fun of it, the charm of it.

In *dhāraṇā,* in the state of *dhāraṇā* or concentration, you have methods and techniques of bringing back the mind. To use the language of Raja Yoga, the mind that was wandering, that was scattered, that was running in ten directions at the same time, hopping from one topic to another, you want to bring it back, and by the concentration of its energies, you want to make it steady. It was disturbed; you would like to make it quiet. It was unsteady; you would like to make it steady.

Concentration is a method of conditioning the mind stuff, the diffused energy. Don't you say that there is the concentrated juice of grapes and then you dilute it? Inside, there is a process of dilution and a process of concentration going on constantly throughout the day. When you allow your attention to wander unnecessarily, unwarrantedly in an irresponsible way, you allow it to wander to hundreds of subjects, the vital energy gets diffused.

Patanjali talks about *dhāraṇā* after *pratyāhāra. Dhāraṇā* is a process of conditioning the mind, conditioning the movement of the past contained in your body, in the nerves, in the chemical system.

How do you condition? There are methods and techniques evolved by Eastern people who have been experimenting in the laboratory of their own bodies for centuries over centuries. As you have been doing with science and technology in the West, and you have helped man to land on the moon, you have helped man to travel in space and be there for months together. As you have conditioned matter to bring back pictures from Neptune, they have been conditioning matter in their bodies, like the breath system in their body, for investigating and exploring the nature of Reality.

In the West, it has been with outward matter, external matter; in the East, it has been with inner matter. Body is matter like the cosmos. It is condensed cosmos. It contains energies, it contains matter, it has the fire principle, the water principle inside it, and there is nothing here that is not there outside. It is a replica on a miniature scale of all that exists in the universe, of all the things that exist in the cosmos—if I may use the term.

You will come across literally hundreds of methods of *dhāraṇā*—concentration. If you turn to Mantra Yoga, they will help you to learn concentration. A mantra yogi who has specialized in sound metaphysics and the handling of sound energy, he can know which kind of sound will be agreeable to your body and your temperament. He can suggest a mantra to you which is a composition of letters, a combination of letters which can be used for quieting your mind, and he will tell you how to repeat it, at what pitch, at what volume, how many times, at what time of day.

These mantra yogis will go into the details of telling you what color clothes you should wear while you are using the mantra. See the specialization! In the West, you have specialized by making those computers where in a tiny silicon chip you can feed in 33,000 pieces of memory, but there you have conditioned outer matter. Here they have conditioned the inside matter. So the mantra yogi has a method. It's not only a ritual. When a mantra yogi asks you to wear pink colored robes or light blue, sky blue clothes or orange colored clothes, it is not a ritual. If the person has studied properly and not just followed the tradition blindly, they can tell you, because it is a science, where with the help of sound you are working upon the energies within your body. For that, you need a technique. Body is matter. The sound energy contained in you, in your body is also matter. You are trying to condition it, and for that you require a method, a technique, and you have to learn it very precisely. The mantra yogi in China, in Tibet, in India won't allow you to speak any way you like. There is a method, mathematical as in Tantra Yoga.

In Tantra Yoga they will teach you postures because they want to change the direction of the sex energy and help the sex energy to travel upward in the body instead of going downward, combining it with pranayama. They want to reverse the direction of the flow of sex energy and take it upward to the crown of the head. That is all Tantra is really about—with the help of pranayama, to reverse the direction of this sex energy. As the sex energy has creative powers, it can create another human being. Look at the potential creativity contained in sex! Sex is something so sacred, so divine, so beautiful. We have dragged it down to only a pleasure level because we are a pleasure-mongering race, a pleasure-obsessed race. But there is the joy, the beauty, the divinity, the sanctity of sex, if only we could understand and appreciate it.

In Tantra Yoga, as we have to study those asanas, the language of chakras, it requires a method, and you must study with the teacher like in Mantra Yoga, like in Hatha Yoga, because you are working upon the matter inside you, which is invisible, which is intangible, which is infinite, which is not like your feet or hands. You can move them as per your wish, as per your will, but here you are working on subtle matter and in order to avoid mistakes, you have to go about it scientifically. So you need a teacher with whom to study, whether it is Hatha Yoga, Tantra Yoga, or Mantra Yoga—as with classical music. You cannot learn it just by videotapes. You may repeat it, but repetition is not the essence of learning, it is a part of learning. You have to go and live with the musician and see how he improvises in classical music.

The techniques and methods, as a part of conditioning, are necessary up to the level of *dhāraṇā.*

If the concentration is not through mantra, if it is not through tantra, maybe somebody asks you to concentrate upon a picture, upon the flame of a candle. In the East, they do it upon the sun, upon the moon or they ask you to concentrate upon the sky, the space. *Akāśa-dhāraṇā* they call it. Concentrating on the formless or concentrating on the form. Do you see the relevance of method and technique from *yama-niyama-āsana-prāṇāyāmā-pratyāhāra* up to *dhāraṇā?* There is a possibility, a scope, and a relevance of methods and techniques because you are trying to condition something, give it a different direction, trying to make the latent manifest, provoking the energies contained in it.

That is how through *dhāraṇā,* through the study of concentration, one can arouse the latent powers, that is to say, the experiences contained in the subconscious and unconscious. What you call the occult and transcendental experiences, they are all contained in you and me, all the experiences that the race has gone through are contained, concealed in you and me. Concentration, *dhāraṇā* can arouse those experiences, it can arouse the latent powers, it can sophisticate your mind, if you really study concentration, whether you do it through a mantra or through a picture or idol or flame.

That study steadies the mind. The mind was scattered and now you are bringing it to one point, you focus yourself on this one point, you give a point to the mind, a time-duration to the mind, and you sit down and concentrate. You may concentrate on your incoming and outgoing breath, you may concentrate upon the movement of thoughts within you. You take some support for steadying the mind. The steady mind has tremendous power. The steadying of the attention develops so many powers. Clairvoyance and clairaudience are powers that come about by the study of *dhāraṇā,* just to give you two examples. Your memory becomes tremendously rich—the power of concentration sharpens the memory, sharpens the perception. When you listen or look, you receive fully because the attention is steady. If you have studied concentration, the result is always a steady attention. When you perceive, there is steadiness, so you take in more things; when you listen, you are steady, so you take in more things. The quality of reception changes with the study of *dhāraṇā.* The quality of retention in memory changes, and the quality of reproduction changes—you reproduce it exactly as it took place. This is possible in the human body.

The study of *dhāraṇā*—concentration—can develop a number of latent powers and also arouse experiences. It is not a surprise that you find techniques and methods given to you for *dhāraṇā,* but it is not meditation. *Dhāraṇā* is not *dhyāna. Dhyāna* is quite different from *dhāraṇā*—it is the next stage.

Dhyāna

First the energy that was diffused gets concentrated, that which was unsteady is made steady, that which was disturbed becomes peaceful. There is a qualitative transformation in receptivity, in attitude, in retention, in reproduction. A qualitative transformation has taken place through *dhāraṇā.* That is why Patanjali recommends it to yoga students to strengthen the mind stuff, to make it vital, vigorous, always energetic. Never is the mind of a yoga student lazy, lethargic, inattentive, distracted, disturbed—it is always alert and attentive.

In the study of Raja Yoga, you do not get stuck there, you do not get blocked there, that is not the culmination, but it can lead to the next step. And the next step is the identification with the mind stuff that has become steady, peaceful, quiet, and beautifully refined, and later, even the identification with that disappears in the state of meditation. In *dhāraṇā,* in concentration, you divided yourself into the person who conditions and that which gets conditioned. You divided yourself in two. You were conditioning—according to a technique and a method—your inner matter; you were working on yourself, on the subtle part of yourself. In the same way, you work upon your body—you clean it, wash it, bathe it, sit it, stand it.

In *dhāraṇā* there is a voluntary inner division for betterment, for development—but the division is still there. In *dhyāna,* the division ends. That identification with the idea of the "Me," the ego ends. We use that as an instrument, just as we use thought as an instrument, as we use the activity of the eyes, the ears, the vocal chords as an instrument—that is a psychophysical activity.

In *dhyāna,* in meditation, there is no activity at all. Meditation is the ending of all voluntary psychophysical activity. Through ending all activity, further exploration takes place; further exploration is not going to take place through the movement of the past. The movement of the conditioning, the techniques, the methods have served their purpose, and they have conditioned the finest possible matter in you, which you call mind. Mind is matter, it is finest matter, and what you call your physical body is gross matter. They are really one and the same—fine and gross, that is the only difference. Ultimately, Raja Yoga says, matter—your body is the materialization of your thought—ultimately it comes to that, but we are not going to that ultimate point this morning. We are saying that, according to Patanjali, *dhyāna* has no method or technique. Up to *dhāraṇā* techniques, methods are necessary, they have a relevance, anyone who says no method, no education, no discipline is necessary—they are indulging in an illusion. Just by listening to talks, reading books, or academically discussing things, transformation doesn't happen. Whether you call it disciplining yourself, educating yourself, conditioning yourself—whatever name you give to that process of education—you have to equip your matter, you have to bring out all your latent sensitivity contained in your matter, so that the heightened, intensified, and deepened sensitivity causes the transformation—the ultimate transformation.

Vimala is open to correction, but as far as she understands Patanjali, up to *dhāraṇā* techniques, methods are recommended, they are prescribed. Through the gateway of Silence, through the gateway of discontinuity of mental movement, through the gateway of the cessation of the thinking process, one is going to get transported into a different orbit of consciousness, a different dimension of consciousness. Meditation, or *dhyāna,* is for the transportation of consciousness into thought-free, time-free, word-free reality, because after *dhyāna* is *samādhi;* according to Patanjali, it is *dhāraṇā-dhyāna-samādhi.* And you might have noticed how Patanjali goes into so much detail about the different kinds of *samādhi—savitarka/nirvitarka samādhi, savicāra/nirvicāra samādhi, sabīja/nirbīja samādhi.*

He goes on describing the different qualities of *samādhi.* A *samādhi* in which you go in and come out, a *samādhi* in which you are still there to experience and come back and tell your experiences to others. It is difficult to verbalize about *samādhi.* You cannot describe *samādhi,* there is no separation between the cosmic and the individual, there it is all one ocean, you can't even verbalize it. Patanjali has gone into many details in different aphorisms describing the qualities of *samādhi.* Suffice it for us this morning that *dhāraṇā,* according to Patanjali, is a necessary step for *dhyāna.*

Dhyāna is the ending of all techniques and methods. *Dhyāna* is ending the concept that you can transform further. You have tried your level best from *yama-niyama* to *dhāraṇā.* Whatever you could do, you have done. So meditation is the phase in which the last effort is to be made, and that last effort is to be effortless and to be methodless, to be techniqueless. The last effort is to put your whole being in the lap of the cosmic energy, as it were. This is figuratively said. Otherwise, you will say "lap of Cosmic Intelligence" and look upon it as a personal god. No, my dear, but Life being poetry, sometimes such expressions escape. When you go to sleep, you don't make any effort, you relax unconditionally. You have so much faith in sleep that it causes complete forgetfulness, you are not afraid of sleep. No effort, no clinging to the center of the "Me" or "not-Me." You don't sleep as a man or woman, you don't sleep as a Hindu or Catholic. All the self-consciousness is gone completely, unconditionally gone. The only difference between sleep and *samādhi* is that in sleep, there is no awareness except for a yogi. In meditation, there is the same unconditional relaxation, total relaxation and complete elimination of the center of the "Me." You don't say, "I am going to sleep." If you make an effort to sleep, you won't sleep, you'll waste the night in effort, so there is a dimension of effortlessness, which is also a dimension of Life. Effort is one dimension and effortlessness is another. Is there any effort in love? Is there any effort in the majesty of innocence? That is why in Silence also there is no effort, not because we do not appreciate the significance of methods and techniques, but they have no relevance here.

So relax into an unconditional effortlessness and let Life operate upon you. Your effortlessness does not mean a void or a blankness or a darkness or an inertia. Please do see this. Meditation is not a state of inertia, it is not a state of passivity, it is not a state of mere void, but when you thus relax unconditionally, you relax totally, then the Supreme Intelligence operates. Meditation is the activation of the most subtle energy of Intelligence. Meditation transports your whole being from the domination of matter, the domination of instincts and impulses, from the domination of thoughts into the orbit of Intelligence, and the perfume of Intelligence is the energy of awareness.

CHAPTER NINE

Prakriti and Purusha

Question: What is *puruṣa* and what is *prakṛti?*

The Yoga philosophy of Patanjali is based on Kapila's Samkhya philosophy. Kapila and the philosophy of Samkhya came before Patanjali and his Raja Yoga. So the whole Raja Yoga philosophy is based on Samkhya of Kapila.

Samkhya talks about *prakṛti,* or nature. Everything is included in *prakṛti*—all matter fine and gross, even what you call your mind, intellect, and thought, because for them, mind is the finest kind of matter. Everything is covered by that one word *prakṛti,* which can be translated into English as "matter and the realm of energy." Matter and the whole cosmic dance of energies is called *prakṛti* by Kapila in the philosophy of Samkhya, and Patanjali seems to accept that.

Samkhya also talks about *puruṣa,* that which is not matter, that which does not move, that which is knowledge itself, that which is light itself, that which is self-effulgent. It is not that *puruṣa* knows. No, *puruṣa* is Knowledge itself, *puruṣa* is Understanding itself.

There is a division of life according to Samkhya between *prakṛti* and *puruṣa*. Patanjali accepts this analysis of Kapila, and he maintains the term *puruṣa* throughout his aphorisms. But the difference is that he talks about matter and then he talks about *puruṣa*—Intelligence.

We will go through the question of *puruṣa* and *prakṛti,* but please see that there is a limit to which I can talk about it, because if you want to understand the whole thing, you have to go back to Samkhya—the twenty-four principles of nature, or *prakṛti,* and then the twenty-fifth is *puruṣa*. If you have some grasp of Samkhya, then it becomes easy for you to understand whether there is one *puruṣa* or individual *puruṣāḥ* as you have asked in your questions.

Prakṛti

Now we will have to pay special attention to the terminology of Kapila and Patanjali. They differentiate *buddhi* from *manas*. *Buddhi* could be translated into English as "intellect." They differentiate *buddhi,* the principle of the intellect, which discriminates, which analyses, from *manas* or mind for which they also use the word *citta*. The *manas* and the *citta* receive impressions brought by the sense organs, collect them, store them, and carry them over to the intellect, or *buddhi*. *Buddhi,* or intellect, unifies these electric impulses received by the brain center. And after unifying them, it interprets them, and there is a response by the sense organs. The electric impulses are carried over to different centers of the brain, and the *buddhi* stands behind them, unifying them, organizing them.

Puruṣa

The second category is what they call *puruṣa,* which has nothing to do with nature, with matter—it is entirely on its own. This *puruṣa,* you can call it the Cosmic Self, you can call it the Seer, the *jñāna,* or the Knowledge, the Understanding. *Puruṣa* is not of matter, *puruṣa* is something unchangeable, nonmaterial, constituted of perception and understanding—that is *puruṣa*.

So you have matter or nature, including mind, on the one hand, and on the other, you have *puruṣa* or Self or *ātma*—sometimes the word *ātman* is also used for the Self, the *puruṣa*.

Here is the nonmaterial, completely separate from the material. They never mix into each other, they are not interchangeable. We are talking about Samkhya philosophy. They are not interconvertible, not interchangeable, they are separate—on their own.

Patanjali, in one of the aphorisms, says, *draṣṭā dṛśi-mātraḥ śuddho'pi pratyaya-anupaśyaḥ* (II.20). *Draṣṭā*—the Seer, the *puruṣa,* the ever-understanding, the ever-intelligent, that Seer is not the doer. It does not do anything. It just is. In our modern parlance, perhaps we could call it the absolute ground of existence. Physics today analyzes life into matter, energy, emptiness behind energy, and the absolute ground of existence behind the emptiness. It analyzes it into these four categories today. According to Samkhya and Kapila and Patanjali, the *puruṣa* is not the doer, the experiencer—it is just the essence of knowledge, the essence of perception.

You have asked me, what is *puruṣa* and what is *prakṛti?* Now if these two—the matter and the Seer, *prakṛti* and *puruṣa*—if they are so independent of each other, so separate of each other, existing side by side, what is the purpose of their existence? Kapila does not provide the answer. He just goes on stating, goes on enumerating the *tattvas* out of which *prakṛti* is constituted and gives a little description of the Seer—the *puruṣa.* But Patanjali proceeds further. And as far as I can understand Patanjali Yoga, he seems to imply that the purpose of nature, of matter is to provide an opportunity for the *puruṣa* to experience his own nature. A very interesting, a very problematic, controversial reply is given by Patanjali Yoga—that the purpose of the whole of existence, the purpose of this innumerable variety of material expressions is to provide an opportunity for the *puruṣa,* for the Seer to experience his separateness from *prakṛti.*

How does that experience take place? If the *puruṣa* is nonmaterial, self-effulgent, completely independent on his own or its own, how does the experience take place if it is for his experience? For that is what Patanjali says, that the purpose of *prakṛti* is for the experience of the *puruṣa,* for the experience of his own nature, for the recognition of his own nature.

Draṣṭṛ-dṛśyayoḥ saṃyogo heya-hetuḥ (II.17)

Draṣṭṛ—Seer; *dṛśya*—that which is seen. The contact between the Seer and the seen, the Seer and that which is seen or experienced, the contact of both is the cause of pleasure and pain. The cause of pleasure and pain, the cause of experience is the contact between the two.

Now we have to find out from our daily life, how the contact takes place. Let us go back, the sense organs are there in the body and there is the contact with the matter outside. It is perceived. The sense organs are matter, the material objects outside are matter, and what is seen is also matter. But the sense organs are finer matter. The sense organs are finer than the trees, the sense organs are finer than the plants. This finer matter gets in touch with the gross matter. That contact creates a sensation. The sensation is possible because there is life in the tree, the tree is not dead; it may be gross and the sense organs may be finer, but it is not dead, there is life in it. Maybe the life is mute, maybe the Intelligence is not as eloquent or as expressive, but it is still there. The sensitivity and consciousness is as much there in the atom as it is in you and me. The nature of the functioning of the sensitivity may be different, but it is still there. Life pervades everything, the Intelligence of creativity permeates everything, and so the contact creates a sensation.

The contact between the finer and the gross takes place and there is a sensation. We saw how it is carried to the still finer—the gray matter in the brain—and behind the brain center is the *buddhi,* or intellect—the unifying principle, still a part of nature, but it is the finest part. Now the *buddhi* as the unifying principle interprets according to its conditioning, according to its *saṃskārāḥ.*

All this is going on within matter. Contact, interaction, involvement, interpretation. And the *puruṣa,* the Seer, the *draṣṭṛ* is alongside this. As it is in the cosmos, so it is in the human body. The same principle—*puruṣa* and *prakṛti,* the Seer and the seen—it is there. That Supreme Intelligence is existing side by side, by his *prakṛti.* The coexistence of the two causes the conjunction in the body, in the material as well as the nonmaterial. It is the coexistence, it is just the coexistence that causes the experience.

Out of the experience, the *puruṣa,* out of ignorance, thinks it suffers pleasure and pain. You have asked me, Where does this *avidyā* come from? I don't know where *avidyā* comes from. I don't want to give you any theories, I don't know how this contact creates *māyā,* the illusion, or how the Intelligence of the Seer gets clouded. It is the perception of the Seer getting clouded which is called *avidyā.* Forgetting its own nature and identifying with the pain or pleasure that is taking place in *prakṛti.*

Draṣṭṛ-dṛśyayoḥ saṃyogo heya-hetuḥ (II.17): The cause of all pleasure and pain is the conjunction of the Seer and that which is seen. The *puruṣa* is the Seer. Instead of just seeing, it has an illusion that "I am experiencing." The movement is going on in *prakṛti,* it is going on in the body, but somehow the Intelligence gets clouded, gets covered up, and the *puruṣa* begins to feel, "I am suffering, I am going through the experience of pain and pleasure."

One of the next aphorisms says, *draṣṭā dṛśi-mātraḥ śuddho'pi pratyaya-anupaśyaḥ* (II.20). *Draṣṭā* is really only "the principle of seeing." *Śuddho—*

"ever pure." And this ever-pure, ever-seeing principle, how does it mistake what is happening in matter as what is happening in him? It is a question unanswered, as far as my perception and understanding goes. It is unanswered not only by Yoga and Samkhya but remains unanswered up to Vedanta. One has studied the six systems of Indian philosophy, and either they say that every experience is painful—*sarvam dukham*—like Gautama the Buddha, or they explain, as Patanjali and Kapila have done, that the conjunction of Seer and the seen causes pain and pleasure. But the question arises, if they are so separate as matter and nonmatter, how does the identification take place?

The origin of *avidyā,* the cause of *avidyā,* according to Patanjali in one of his aphorisms, is *tasya hetur-avidyā* (II.24). Ignorance is the cause of suffering. Where does the ignorance come from? They don't know. Modern seers like Krishnamurti say it is a wrong question. Whether it is a wrong question or a right question, I have to confess my ignorance, I do not know the origin of *avidyā,* or ignorance. I know it is there only because we have experienced it in ourselves. When the movement of pleasure and pain takes place in the body, when the movement of pleasure and pain takes place in the thought stream, somehow there is identification, and you feel that you are enjoying or suffering.

The whole science of yoga is to enable a student to discriminate between *puruṣa* and *prakṛti,* to discriminate between the movement of thought, which is a movement of ideas, and become aware that pain and pleasure take place in matter, that it is a movement in matter. Thinking, feeling, willing is a movement that takes place in matter. Thought is matter, but that which recognizes matter as matter seems to be independent of it, and therefore there is no pain in Intelligence. Whether you call it *puruṣa* or you do not call it *puruṣa,* it is your and my experience that some principle registers the happenings, registers that happening of pain, registers the happening of pleasure—obviously it must be independent of the movement of pleasure and pain. If it is not independent of the movement, if it is not the Seer of the movement, if it is not independent of the experience of pain and pleasure, it could not register it, it could not verbalize it, it could not evaluate it.

Whether in the language of Kapila or Patanjali or in our own language of modern science, we can say there seems to be a principle of Intelligence, an ever-seeing principle in the cosmos and within ourselves which creates a harmony in nature and which enables us to discriminate between the happenings outside and the ever-seeing principle inside.

Draṣṭā and *dṛśya*—the Seer and the seen, they seem to be two categories. Intelligence does not change. Intellect changes, thought changes, thought can get affected by forgetfulness. So intellect, thought, feelings, they are changing principles, they are in the orbit of matter, but Intelligence, Awareness, Love, Compassion do not change. Whether they are the constituents of *puruṣa,* I don't know. I don't know whether to call him *puruṣa* or not to call him *puruṣa,* but there definitely seems to be an all-permeating, omnipotent, omniscient, omnipresent energy of Intelligence incorporated in everything and therefore incorporated also in us.

This is rather abstruse and abstract, but Patanjali Yoga has its part of abstract philosophy and mental discipline, just as it has a practical, concrete aspect of yama, niyama, etc.

The significant point of difference between all the Eastern religions and our modern science of physics, etc., is this: according to the East, from the Supreme Principle of Intelligence, from the *puruṣa,* from the Seer, the whole creation has exploded, and in the West, according to modern science, it is matter getting finer and finer, and then the principle of consciousness evolving, developing, becoming self-expressive. So Intelligence comes last. The Eastern religions say just the opposite. They say first there was *caitanya—sat-cit-ānanda.* There was the indestructible Truth—*sat;* spontaneous Understanding—*cit;* and causeless Bliss—*ānanda.* They say there was this principle of *sat-cit-ānanda,* out of which came the world. So Intelligence comes first, according to them, which they call the *mahat,* and according to science it comes last. But wherever you begin, the principle of Intelligence gets involved. You call it the Supreme Intelligence because you think it comes last. So it is very difficult for a European or an American or a non-Indian to get the feel of, to get hold of what Kapila and Patanjali want to say about *puruṣa* and *prakṛti.* I can appreciate the difficulty any of you may have felt about it.

If you go back from Yoga, from Samkhya to the Vedas, go back to the first Veda, the Rig Veda, in the tenth mantra there is a sutra in which the Seer says that before the cosmos exploded out of Life, or Is-ness, everything was undifferentiated, nonindividuated. You could not differentiate truth from untruth. There was nothing that you could call day, nothing that you could call night. You could not differentiate death from life and birth. There was such a nebulous condition of existence—undifferentiated, unindividuated. Only an ocean of Intelligence, but nondifferentiated. That is what they say in Rig Veda.

And then you come to Samkhya, where they analyze matter and nonmatter, matter and spirit, soul, self, or *ātman*—so many terms have been used. That analysis is there and then the question of their relationships is there—why and how the conjunction takes place, what the conjunction causes—the experience of pain and pleasure.

And then the science of Yoga says you have to go through the experience of pleasure and pain. The pain and pleasure take place in matter. You have to go back to your virgin, pristine purity, you are only the Seer of it—*draṣṭā dṛśi-mātraḥ śuddho'pi pratyaya-anupaśyaḥ* (II.20). They are happenings only in the gross matter, they don't affect you. You are neither the sinner nor the saint. You are the ever-pure Seer beyond experiencing. All these terms can make anyone dizzy unless you study the whole Eastern approach to cosmogenesis, the evolution, etc.

For our understanding of Patanjali, *puruṣa* is the principle of Supreme Intelligence that is a perceptive sensitivity. That Intelligence has inbuilt the quality of perception, of understanding. Perception, understanding is not its activity, it is its quality. The understanding is built in, it is within us. So while we go through the experiences of pain and pleasure, it is possible to learn not to identify with them and through that nonidentification to be aware that we are the other, that we are not the body, we are not the thoughts, we are not the pain, that we are independent of the happenings in the body, we are the other, which is the essence of our being. This is only the crust, up to the mind it is the crust, up to the interpretations by the brain and the conditioning, it is only the crust. But the essence, the Lifeness of our being is the ever-seeing Intelligence. I have no other word.

Question: Is there one *puruṣa* or are there individual *puruṣāḥ?*

The soul, the *puruṣa* is in each one of us, that Supreme Intelligence exists in each one of us. If you would like to call it individual *puruṣa,* you may call it individual *puruṣa,* because it is sheltered in the human body, as a pearl is sheltered in a shell.

The *puruṣa,* that cosmic principle of Intelligence, the Seer, the *draṣṭā* is encased in the body along with matter. So if you like to call it individual *puruṣa,* you can call it individual *puruṣa.* It is like the ray of sunlight. If you like to say that this ray that has come in my room has individuality, you may say that, but it comes from the sun, it originates there and it goes back there. In the same way, as soon as a child is born, there is this principle of Supreme Intelligence, the Seer, the *draṣṭā* inside the body. Call it individual if you want to. Patanjali accepts calling it individual *puruṣa,* originating from the ultimate *puruṣa,* from the *paramadraṣṭā.* The individual—*vyakti draṣṭā* and the cosmic—the *paramadraṣṭā.* The principle of *draṣṭuḥ*—seeing and seeingness is the same in both.

Question: If *puruṣa* permeates everything, then all the atoms of my body, all the atoms in the air around me are permeated by *puruṣa.* I cannot understand how there is an individual *puruṣa* that is not of this body, of this Earth! If *puruṣa* is in every atom in me and without me, then what difference is there between the *puruṣa* of the atoms and individual *puruṣa?*

No difference. In essence, there is no difference. You call it individual because you feel the Intelligence here in the body. It is a figurative way of speaking, but it is an undifferentiated and unindividuated, all-permeating principle of Intelligence. Really, *puruṣa* is neither imprisoned in the body nor a completely separate entity—that idea comes later on in the Indian mythology of jivas. All that language comes later on. Up to Patanjali, up to that point, it was not distorted or twisted.

One has to watch and find out what is matter in us, how it functions, how the conditioning functions, and what is the Seer, due to whose presence this observation becomes possible. It's an ancient science and an ancient philosophy.

Question: Are *puruṣa* and *prakṛti* a duality?

Yes, according to Samkhya, they are a duality and the two remain separate. Patanjali accepts the duality but qualifies it.

Soul, self, *ātman*—all these terms are used for *puruṣa,* and for cosmos they use the terms *paramātman, brahman, paramapuruṣa.*

Because the body is individuated, the Intelligence inhabiting the body was looked upon as being individuated, differentiated, separated. You were right in asking if it permeates the whole universe, how can it be looked upon as individuated, becoming an entity inside the body? It can't, but that was the way of presenting, of explaining things in 553 B.C.

Question: I cannot understand how *draṣṭā* and *puruṣa* are the same thing.

Draṣṭā is the description of the *puruṣa. Draṣṭā* means "Seer." *Puruṣa* is *draṣṭā.* It is called *puruṣa* because the whole cosmos is a shell. *Puraṃ* is a Sanskrit word from which the word *puruṣa* is derived. *Puraṃ* is the shell, the whole cosmos is a big shell in which dwells that principle of *puruṣa. Puruṣa*—that which dwells in a shell. For the cosmos, the word used is *brahmānda. Aṇḍa* is egg. It looks like a big egg. Sometimes they call it *hiraṇyagarbha*, they call it *virata.* That which dwells in the shell of the cosmos is *puruṣa.* To differentiate the shell and that which inhabits it, they use the term *puruṣa.* That is a romantic way of putting these things.

Now what is this *puruṣa,* what does he do? *Draṣṭā*—he is ever-seeing. Not the experiencer, just the Seer. They don't call him only a witness, they don't say, "He is only a witness"; they say, "He is the Seer." And how is that seeing? That seeing includes and involves understanding. Perception and understanding are blended together. So you cannot differentiate the two, you cannot say that the seeing takes place and then a fraction of second later the understanding takes place. They say they are blended into one—two in one. So *puruṣa* is *draṣṭā* and the *jñānatatva* both. The Seer and the Understanding both.

The whole universe is *dṛśya. Dṛśya* is that which is seen. The Sanskrit root from which the word *darśana* comes means "to see." In describing Indian philosophy you hear the word *darśana. Darśana*—singular and *darśanāni* —plural. The six systems of Indian philosophy are called *darśanāni.* That which has been seen and understood is Darshan philosophy.

Question: You said earlier that the *puruṣa,* the Seer identifies with the pleasure and pain and the thought, but how does the Seer, which is not thought, identify with thought, because "I am suffering" is a thought.

My dear, did I not say I do not know where this basic ignorance originates, how this confusion comes about, which is called *mūla avidyā.*

What is the cause of this conjunction of Seer and the seen, *draṣṭā* and *dṛśya?* Patanjali says, *tasya hetur-avidyā* (II.24): Ignorance is the cause. Where does the ignorance come from? We don't know. Since the evolution of the human race, human beings have mistaken the experiences taking place, the changes taking place in matter as happening within the Seeing Principle. There has been this confusion.

If we want to find out how it happened, we will have to observe it in ourselves. For example, when there is a toothache or a headache, don't I say, "I have pain." Not figuratively, but literally, I feel that I am in pain. If the "I" is not the tooth, not the head, and the pain is taking place in the head, how does the identification take place? Because I feel that "I" am the body, the identification is taken for granted. You and I were brought up that way, we grew up with this idea. How did it happen in the beginning of society? How did it happen with the first human being? I do not know, but this identification seems to be there, taken for granted.

Question: Is thinking a property of *buddhi* or *manas?*

Of both. *Buddhi* discriminates, interprets. Mind collects.

Again let, me clarify I am talking about Patanjali. I am talking about Samkhya and Patanjali Yoga. Next week, if you ask me, my answer could be different. Please do see this. I am sitting here to explain what this philosophy means. Vimala is not sitting here to talk about her understanding of life. She is sitting here as a teacher would sit in a class to talk about Raja Yoga, which is a philosophy of Patanjali. So with great respect I share my understanding of those aphorisms. That is why I said earlier, please don't think that I agree with everything that every aphorism says.

Eastern philosophers and sages have analyzed the mind stuff. They have analyzed it down to the finest possible matter, to the minutest degree possible, as far as they can possibly reach. They have given four different names to the functions of the mind stuff: *manas, buddhi, citta, ahaṃkāra.*

Collecting agency is the mind—*manas.* (Memorizing, which is different from collecting, is *smṛti.*)

Retaining agency is *citta.*

Analyzing agency is *buddhi.*

And *ahaṃkāra* is the monitor of all these.

Question: Would *citta vṛtti nirodhaḥ* mean *buddhi vṛtti nirodhaḥ?*

Yes. It is really, my friend, transcending the illusion of being the experiencer of pain and pleasure. That is all there is to this business of Raja Yoga and its mental disciplines.

You are not the experiencer, nor the doer. It is the *prakṛti* that is the doer, that is the experiencer.

You—the essence of your being—are only the Seer, the Seer-ness. That is how I understand the essence of Raja Yoga.

CHAPTER TEN

Raja Yoga and the Art of Living

If you have taken the journey with the speaker so far, you might have noticed that Raja Yoga is a science of Life and simultaneously an art of living. As a science of Life, it analyses the wholeness of Life, it analyzes the cosmogenesis and tells us in very clear terms that just as a spider weaves a net around itself out of the substance of its own body, *puruṣa,* the Supreme Intelligence, a fountain of an inexhaustible potential of creativity, manifests, or rather, weaves, what you call a cosmos around itself out of the substance of its own being.

The being of the *puruṣa,* the ever-seeing Intelligence, the ever-sensitive creativity manifests itself first in the principle that is called *mahat.* That is to say, the principle of Intellect where the *sattva, rajas,* and *tamas*—the faculty of knowing, the faculty of activity, and the potential of inertia—are in a state of spontaneous balance.

Mahat is the finest expression, perhaps the first manifestation of what could be called matter, what could be called *prakṛti.* When the equipoise gets disturbed, that is to say, the *sattva, rajas,* and *tamas* begin to play around with themselves and the ratio of their quantity and quantum begins to fluctuate, then out of the *mahat* comes the ten *mātra.*

From the *ātman,* from the *puruṣa,* from the *caitanya,* from the Supreme Intelligence, the first manifestation is *ākāśa.*

From *ākāśa,* the second manifestation comes as *prāṇa*—the vital energy.

Prāṇa explodes into what you call *agni*—in the form of suns and moons and the heat around us.

From *agni,* from that principle of fire, manifests water, which seems to be contradictory.

From water, or *āpa,* earth is generated.

From earth, or *pṛthivī,* the cereals, the grains, etc., are generated, which feed and sustain the *prāṇī,* or the creatures with *prāṇa*—birds, animals, human beings.

As a science of Life, it gives us the cosmogenesis of what we call the universe. There may be millions of such universes. We may be aware only of this tiny universe that we live in with its solar systems and planets.

To put it in a different way, as a science of Life, Patanjali's Yoga describes to us how matter exploded out of *puruṣa.* I'm not referring to Sankhya this morning. We are focusing our attention only on Patanjali and Patanjali's Yoga—all the references to the background and foundation in Sankhya have been talked about.

So there is that nonmaterial Intelligence, the Cosmic Intelligence that is called *puruṣa,* and then the explosion of matter—gradual and systematic. One element coming after the other logically—first the finest, then the less fine, then the two categories of *prakṛti,* or matter, and then the ever-shining, ever-sensitive Seer or *puruṣa,* the Supreme Intelligence which never gets affected by the movement that takes place in matter.

Though the matter has exploded out of the substance of *caitanya,* just as the web is formed by the spider, but the spider remains independent of the net that he weaves around himself, the *puruṣa,* the *caitanya,* the *ātman* remain unaffected by what happens in matter.

Now this explosion of matter from *ākāśa* to *vāyu* to *agni* to *āpa* to *pṛthivī,* etc., is nothing but interaction of innumerable energies.

Intelligence, or *puruṣa,* as we saw, is a fountain of an inexhaustible potential of energy. Millions of universes have exploded out of the fountain, that ground of existence, that *satta,* that *caitanya,* and yet the creativity remains inexhaustible.

The creativity contained in that Supreme Intelligence is shared by what you call the *ākāśa,* the *manas,* and matter up to the grossest possible particle of atom, proton, electron of matter. The creativity is shared by matter. As it has exploded out of *caitanya,* it contains the energy of creativity. Therefore neither the *ākāśa,* the so-called emptiness of space, nor the earth, which looks so solid, can be called dead matter. They are gross forms of creative energy, they are the result of interactions of unknown and perhaps innumerable energies.

So here is matter and inside that matter is what you call mind—the thought stream. Thought is a name given to one of the energies that human beings have discovered in matter, within matter. Now we human beings are born within it, and we ourselves are composed of fine matter and gross matter. We are constituted of innumerable energies, which are solidified and we call them matter. Please do see this. The whole material world is really a field of interplay and interaction of energy. When they are solidified, you call them matter; when they are nonsolidified, you call them energy. When they are not individuated, when they are not differentiated, then you call them space, emptiness, or *ākāśa*. And beyond the emptiness of space or *ākāśa* remains the fountain, the absolute ground of existence, the *puruṣa*.

The *puruṣa* and the *prakṛti* exist in you and me on a tiny scale. They exist in the Earth in a bigger form, in the universe on a still wider and bigger scale. So the interplay of energies goes on, and the Intelligence shines behind the interplay of energies—solidified, nebulous, differentiated, undifferentiated—that is the dance of Shiva, that is the cosmic dance of Life, that goes on. This is Patanjali's analysis of what Life is.

He tells us this, after he must have investigated, experimented, explored in his body. The Upanishads, the Vedas, all the six systems of Indian philosophy are not mere or sheer literature, they are not creations out of imagination, they are not fiction—they are the result of explorations, experimentations gone through by those, our ancestors. They are the ancestors not only of the Indians, they are the ancestors of the whole human race—Patanjali, Kapila, or the seers of the Upanishads, who were analyzing what Life is which was their tremendous interest.

What does the seer Patanjali want us to do after he has given this philosophy to us, which I'm putting very briefly? Why does he want us to know this? In order that we the humans who are born with an evolved consciousness can be free of bondage.

Freedom from Ignorance—Avidyā

The energy of creativity in us is not mute, as in the mineral world. It is not as mute as in the animals or in the kingdom of the birds, it has the faculty of self-awareness. We can look at ourselves mentally. We can introspect, retrospect; there is this capacity of self-awareness that enables us to observe, to watch, to analyze, to understand.

Patanjali says that the goal of human life, the purpose of human life is to understand the nature of Reality, to understand the role of matter, to understand the role of energies, and to understand the essence of Intelligence. It is only understanding that liberates; it is ignorance that binds. We human beings feel that we are in bondage, that we are slaves of matter, that we are prisoners of mind and thought. To them, Patanjali says there is no slavery, there is no prison-house, it is only ignorance.

Tasya hetur-avidyā (II.24). There is only ignorance about the nature of matter, about what you call mind, and about the source of Life—the *puruṣa*, or the Intelligence.

Freedom from Attachment—Rāga

Now take the second step with Patanjali, who says that what you call matter, or energy, is always changing. It is always in flux. It cannot remain idle, it cannot remain static. Matter is always changing. What you call your body, the gross form, is changing. Not only every day, perhaps every hour, and if you go to the finest particle within you, perhaps every minute. In the quality of blood, in the quality of cells, there is constant change going on. Birth is the beginning of the flux of change, of the torrent of change.

Witness the changes taking place in the matter in you, and you will understand the constant flux that is taking place. Knowing that life around you, on the material level in which you are living is a huge torrent of change, do not try to arrest that, do not try to impose a theory or permanency on that.

Come to the less gross layer of your being, where you have sense organs. The capacity of the sense organs also grows, decays, and disintegrates, just as the gross matter of the body grows, decays, and disintegrates. The eyes that can see very sharply in childhood may and can become dim in old age. The power of hearing may get affected, the sense organs with their faculties also are going to change. So do not get attached to the experience that sight gives you, because they are also going to change their nature as the body grows old. Enjoy while you are in the prime of youth.

Patanjali does not say run away from experiences. He says to let every experience be the opportunity for self-discovery, let every experience be an occasion to find out what is an experience and who is the experiencer that is experiencing. Experiences are an occasion of liberation, they are opportunities for self-discovery. That is the thing I have learned from Patanjali.

You need not deny pleasure. When the sense organs come into touch with their respective objects, enjoy the pleasure they give. Go through that sensation, but never get attached, because you are in a field of flux. Attachment will begin the cycle of misery and suffering. The world is made for enjoyment, the sense organs are given to you with the sensitivity to enjoy, but enjoyment knows no attachment. Go through the experience with alertness, with sensitivity, understanding that experiences take place in the timelessness of Life. Do not try to impose your psychological time, to give it continuity, and say "I had it this morning, I must have it tomorrow." It is only when you introduce the factor of psychological time in the orbit of enjoyment—which is the result of communication of the energy of your sense organs and the energy of the matter around you—that suffering, or misery, begins. Otherwise there is nothing like misery and suffering.

We are talking about the art of living, so do not impose any theories on this constant flux of change, the vortex of change in which we are born and with which we have to live. Do not get attached to any expression of matter, fine or gross. Whether you get attached to others—or you get attached to the qualities of the mind like virtue or feel repulsion against vice—it is all going to cause misery, because there is nothing permanent in the orbit of matter and energy. Change is the Reality and every theory about permanence is an idea.

Freedom from Abhiniveśa

Proceed still further: to the energy layer of your being which you call the realm of *manas, citta, buddhi, ahaṃkāra.* The whole thought stream, and its movement in you and the memory in you, is your inheritance. Most of it is inheritance not from the family but from the whole human race. You are the condensed human past. You have that thought stream with you—it is composed of impressions contained in your blood, in your bones, in your flesh, and it is constantly changing.

There is constant change, and therefore it would be stupidity to impose the idea of permanency, an idea of continuity, on that thought structure.

We call it "thought stream," "thought structure." We are using the words, but there is nothing like permanency and nothing like continuity in Life. That is the beauty of Life, and then there comes the moment of dying. Disintegration of forms—they are being burned down, they are being buried, getting one with the earth, and then again taking new forms. Emergence of forms in matter and merging back into the formlessness—the dance of Shiva goes on; Life is a flux. *Avidyā* causes misery. *Asmitā,* believing that there is an ego and creating egoism out of it, causes suffering. Attachment and repulsion, *rāga* and *dveṣa,* cause suffering, and so does *abhiniveśa*—clinging to life.

There is a beautiful sutra given by Patanjali—*avidyā-asmitā-rāga-dveṣa-abhiniveśāḥ kleśāḥ* (II.3).

Harmonious Living

Patanjali takes you a step further. Holding your hand, he takes you a step further and says, "If you remember the whole of creation is an emergence out of the substance of that Intelligence, of that Creativity, you will see that the whole of Life is one, it is a wholeness, it is an organic wholeness, it is homogeneous wholeness, and therefore, in the art of living, be aware of it."

Ahiṃsā-satya-asteya-brahmacarya-aparigrahā yamāḥ (II.30). The guiding light of the yamas will help you not to get attached, not to get stuck, as will the attitude of noninjury. You are a part of Life, and as in an ocean, where every drop is related to every other, we are related to each other. We are related to the animals and birds, to the trees, the mountains, the rivers. We are related to one another. We feel we are separate because we don't see the mass of space that has connected us. In space are innumerable energies which keep you and me interrelated and interconnected. We have forgotten the connection, that interrelatedness, and therefore we are violent. After inhabiting the planet for many centuries, we have not yet gotten over even that barbaric violence in us! Patanjali says to cultivate *ahiṃsā*—noninjury—as an art of living for being in harmony with the cosmic life.

The yamas are necessary. We do not want to go into them again, but from noninjury right up to nonpossessiveness, this is the key of living in harmony.

What we have to do is to live in harmony with one another and with the nonhuman species, with the whole cosmos. Harmony is the proof of Intelligence. Thought can create disharmony, thought can create comparison, jealousy. Intelligence leads toward harmony and cooperation. Thought wants to assert. Intelligence is fulfilled in being. The manifestation of Intelligence is in love, cooperation, harmony—what you call friendship.

So Patanjali Yoga is an education in the psychology of cooperation instead of a psychology of confrontation, a psychology of nonviolence instead of aggression.

How do we do that, how can there be this attitude of noninjury, truthfulness, nonstealing, nonpossessiveness?

Patanjali gives the answer to that question in his aphorism *śauca-santoṣa-tapaḥ-svādhyāya-īśvara-praṇidhānāni niyamāḥ* (II.32). Look at the scientific, the very pragmatic, realistic way of purification!

How do we attain purification? Do the asanas and pranayama to purify the body, and purify the mind by a noncomparative approach, so there will be *śauca-santoṣa*.

Where will I get the strength to do *tapas*? What is *tapas*? As soon as you investigate and understand something, live it immediately, don't allow any time between understanding and the living of that understanding. That is *tapas,* and so on—he shows the way.

But we are to proceed further, because even after purifying through asanas and pranayama, after having become aware of *ahiṃsā-satya-asteya-brahmacarya-aparigrahā,* there is one more important and very significant thing that is extremely necessary, and that is *pratyāhāra.*

Pratyāhāra

Raja Yoga is the science of moderation, self-restraint. It does not talk about giving up the world, it does not talk about the cult of indulgence, it does not mention the cult of suppression or repression. Neither renunciation nor indulgence. It is a science of moderation, of self-restraint, which Buddha called *madhyama mārga*—the Middle Path. Buddha referred to it in a beautiful way, in his own way, as *maitrī, karuṇā, muditā, upekṣā,* which Patanjali also refers to later on in his aphorisms. Buddha took *maitrī, karuṇā, muditā, upekṣā* and based his whole Middle Path on that. You might have read about it. The Hinayana and the Mahayana Buddhists, they talk about it.

Pratyāhāra is the art of moderation. Self-restraint, moderation creates order and orderliness. Excess is ugliness. If you underfeed the body, if you starve it, if it is not given proper nutrition, then there is ugliness, and if you feed it excessively, then again there is ugliness. Excess on both sides creates ugliness, because it creates distortions. In excessiveness is imbalance, and in imbalance is impurity. *Śuddhi-karaṇe saṃtulanam*—purification is the mystery of equipoise and equibalance.

In the chapter on *samādhi*, Patanjali refers to the elimination of *aśuddhi*—elimination of impurities. So moderation keeps you rooted, grounded, where there is no excess either way, neither underfeeding nor overfeeding, undersleeping nor oversleeping, underexercising nor overexercising. You know that excess leads to imbalance, and imbalance is impurity. Imbalance in every action creates a psychic knot. Like a blood clot, there is a psychic clot with every imbalance. With every impurity, there is a clot in the psyche, as it were, and therefore Patanjali talks about *pratyāhāra*.

What is *pratyāhāra?* Very briefly, the sense organs biologically are incorporated in your material body in such a way that they run toward their respective objects. When there is the slightest presence of an object around them, immediately they get attracted toward the outer object, to meet the respective object of their own energies. In the eyes is the energy of sight, so as soon as you are awake and the eyes open, the sight runs through the eyes toward some object. The ears run toward some sound. That is how they are conditioned to get related to material objects around them and bring in sensations. Sense organs seem to be living by collecting sensations.

Now here comes the education in *pratyāhāra*. In *pratyāhāra* you educate each sense organ. You do not expose your ears to aggressive sounds or excessive talk. You hear the words of others or your own sound if and when necessary, and when it is not necessary, there is no excessive talking, even to yourself.

Teaching yourself moderation—moderation in speech, moderation in audition, moderation in perception, moderation in eating, etc. Moderation is not taking vows. It is not a prison-house of musts and must-nots, oughts and ought-nots, which may be so in Hatha Yoga, which may be so in Mantra Yoga or Tantra Yoga. But in Raja Yoga, which is the science of

Life and art of living, there are no musts and must-nots, there are no rigid frameworks to which you have to bind yourself. Because as soon as you bind yourself to some code of conduct, to some discipline, you are denying the creativity of Intelligence within you, and we have to be aware of the potential creativity of Intelligence within us. So we need not build up defense mechanisms, codes of conduct, patterns of behavior and get attached to them, have a vested interest in them, become victimized by them, talking about virtue and sin, talking about heaven and hell. Patanjali does not talk in this way at all. He says that if you once learn moderation—that beautiful art of never doing anything in excess, doing every act precisely, mathematically, scientifically from morning to evening—then excessiveness will not create imbalance or impurities.

That is one thing, and the second thing is that this moderation helps you to conserve energy. Please do see this. The energy is wasted when you do things in an undisciplined way. If we don't provide sufficient sleep to the body, then we are adding an inertia, an imbalance. If we don't sleep at the time we ought to sleep, then we are wasting energy. If we talk too much, we are wasting energy.

Please do see this. Moderation saves us from imbalances and impurities, and moderation results in the conservation of vital energy, which is necessary for meditation. To break through the shell of thought and the ego, to go beyond matter, to go beyond thought, which is the subtlest possible matter, vitality and passion are necessary. Much energy, much vitality is necessary, and for that, energy has to be conserved. *Pratyāhāra* is the source of conservation of energy. It is the key.

Dhāraṇā

All right, we have done it, we have brought moderation in relationship to the body and in relationship to material needs. How do we bring in moderation when it comes to mind? So proceed with Patanjali and go to *dhāraṇā*. The study of *dhāraṇā* teaches moderation toward what you call your mind, which wanders. It wanders over hundreds of places. Through the study of *dhāraṇā,* you give it one direction, whether you give it the direction of the lotus of your heart or the lotus on the crown of your head or you give it the direction of your navel point, you create a direction for it. It is educated to run in one direction. And so that it does not run in that direction endlessly, you give it a point of destination. You give it the idea of God through some picture, some idol, you give it some mantra.

So for conditioning the mind, the thought movement, for bringing it to moderation, you teach it *dhāraṇā*. You give it one direction, one point of destination and teach it to be steady. The ever-wandering, the ever-hopping, the ever-restless mind learns to be steady. It is now brought from many to one. Instead of endlessly wandering, it is now going to one point of destination. You choose the point of destination, says Patanjali, whether you do it through Bhakti Yoga or Mantra Yoga. It does not matter. Take the help of anything that you like, but through the study of *dhāraṇā* make it steady.

Patanjali says, *abhyāsa vairāgyābhyāṃ tan-nirodhaḥ* (I.12). Through *abhyāsa*—study—if you persevere, if you persist, then even when you are working throughout the day, the mind will remain steady, because it has learned steadiness. So the restlessness has disappeared and a new quality, a new faculty of steadiness has come. Whenever it wants to deal with something, the mind will deal with it totally, not in a halfhearted way, not in a distracted, absentminded way, but it will be there totally present, because through concentration, through *dhāraṇā,* you have taught it to be so.

Dhyāna

It is only when the restless mind, the ever-disturbed, ever-divided mind, becomes steady and undivided that it is possible to proceed to *dhyāna*—and then to the entrance into *samādhi.* The word *entrance* does not satisfy me, rather the growth into the dimension of *samādhi,* which is the dimension of the Supreme Intelligence, ever-effulgent, ever-creative.

Patanjali says the destiny of man is to grow into an awareness of the essence of his being, which is the *puruṣa,* which is the Intelligence, which is the creativity. Matter is the shell. Within the matter, within the shell of thought, knowledge, or experience, is the ever-shining, the ever-effulgent perceiver, ever-seeing, ever-knowing—and you are that, says Patanjali.

It is a question of letting go the hold of addiction, of letting go the hold of *avidyā*—ignorance.

To be with matter—its pain, its pleasure, its birth, its death, its flux of change. Being in the midst of it, being aware all the time that you are the Other, the nonmaterial, encased in matter yet qualitatively different.

Raja Yoga is the science of Life and art of living, and the secret of moderation is the source of harmony. No compulsions, no rigidity, no stiff structures or frameworks, but a call to probe your own Intelligence, to dig within yourself and arrive at the source of that Intelligence in yourself as well as in the universe around you.

Awareness of the nature of Reality, purification of the material encasement, which gets dirty every minute, which is changing every minute, so the need for education in keeping it pure. Not that you have purified it once and it will remain pure by itself. It is matter, it has to be cleaned every day, just as the body has to be cleaned every day. Water cleanses the body and Silence cleanses the mind. You bathe it in Silence, you soak it in the emptiness of Silence, and it comes out clean again, fresh for the ordeal and travail of the day.

Awareness of the nature of life, purification as the source of illumination, moderation in our psychophysical movement as the source of conservation of energy, and *samādhi* as the dimension free of all psychological suffering.

Tataḥ kleśa-karma-nivṛttiḥ (IV.30). The purpose of studying Patanjali Yoga is the ending of psychological misery and suffering. *Kleśāḥ-nivrttiḥ* is the term used by Patanjali. You might study Yajnavalkya Smriti—the conclusion would be the same. You might turn to Shvetashvatara Upanishad, which also talks about yoga. The same conclusion about *kleśāḥ-nivrttiḥ* would be there.

CHAPTER ELEVEN

Purification

Sattva-puruṣayoḥ śuddhi-sāmye kaivalyam-iti (III.56)

We saw yesterday that Raja Yoga is the science of life and living. It is a holistic science encompassing the totality of life. We saw how it analyzes life and gives the genesis of the cosmos by indicating that *puruṣa,* the Supreme Intelligence, is the source of life. In *puruṣa,* or that absolute ground of existence, is seeing-ness, or unconditional Intelligence; knowing-ness, or unconditional Understanding; being-ness, or inexhaustible Creativity; all blended together.

Along with *puruṣa,* Patanjali teaches us about matter and goes into a very elaborate analysis of matter at all the levels and all the layers—from the grossest possible to the finest possible form of matter. He analyzes the solidified matter and the nonsolidified matter which is energy. He analyzes the vibrational forms of energy and the potential form of energy. It is marvelous how he goes through the analysis of matter, mind, and intellect. Patanjali Yoga uses one word to describe all this—*prakṛti.*

We saw yesterday how purification, moderation, and transformation are suggested by Patanjali as a way of living. It is a way of living in the same absolute freedom and sensitivity that *puruṣa,* or the source of life, exists.

In the last few days, we have just been touching the fringes of Raja Yoga. It is a vast, all-encompassing, all-inclusive, holistic science. It is impossible to look at Raja Yoga elaborately, intensively, comprehensively in one week or even one month—it demands and it requires a long study.

If what we saw yesterday is clear to both the listeners and the speaker, we will look at that science of life this morning, the last morning together, from a different angle.

Yoga is a science of purification and transformation, and the purification has to begin at the point of perception. Patanjali analyzes the mechanism of perception very beautifully. The mechanism of sensory perception, extrasensory perception, mental perception, supramental perception, and so on. In his inimitable, elegant way, he analyzes the mechanism of purification. And for the purification of the physical, you have to begin at the sense organ level.

The purification of the sensory has to take place, and for that he suggests asana and pranayama. For the purification of the mental, he suggests yama and niyama; for the purification of the extrasensory, he suggests the study of *dhāraṇā.* And for transformation in the whole content of the sensory, extrasensory, and mental, he suggests *dhyāna,* or meditation. And with the culmination of this process of purification into *dhyāna,* or meditation, descends *samādhi,* or the transformed consciousness, and that is the last phase.

The dimension in which Patanjali expects human beings to live is *samādhi. Samādhi* as the dimension of consciousness and dynamics of relationship, the culmination of the first seven limbs of Ashtanga Yoga: *yama-niyama-āsana-prāṇāyāma-pratyāhāra-dhāraṇā-dhyāna*—all culminating in the awakening of *samādhi.*

We have the purification of the sensory, the purification of the mental, the purification of the extrasensory, and the awakening of the supramental—of the transformed consciousness.

Sattva-puruṣayoḥ śuddhi-sāmye kaivalyam-iti (III.56)

Raja Yoga is for enabling human beings to live in the state of *kaivalyam,* the absolute, unconditional freedom, absolute unconditional sensitivity that could be called love and compassion.

A great giant, Shri Aurobindo, talks about Raja Yoga as Integral Yoga. He has divided Ashtanga Yoga into two parts—*yama-niyama-āsana-prāṇāyāma* for the ascent of matter, as he calls it, and *pratyāhāra-dhāraṇā-dhyāna-samādhi* for the descent of the supramental. It is a beautiful way in which he has analyzed Integral Yoga. You must have heard about Aurobindo, who has written about the Vedas. His approach to the Vedas, his interpretation of Gita, is based upon his own yogic experiences, and his main contribution to Indian culture and the world human culture is the work that he calls Integral Yoga. The ascent of matter and descent of the Divine. That is his language. Every inquirer and explorer of the Divine in India has his or her own unique way. But no one has until now arrived at the dimension of *samādhi* without passing through Raja Yoga. This seems to be an inevitable avenue of purification, illumination, transformation, which every inquirer has to pass through.

We are going to look this morning at this aphorism: *sattva-puruṣayoḥ śuddhi-sāmye kaivalyam-iti* (III.56).

As I said, we have touched only the fringes, not even the whole periphery. Though you may try to do it briefly, it is a very complex, very rich, and all-inclusive approach to life, with so many nuances, so many shades of meaning, elaborated scientifically, poetically. The beauty of Raja Yoga is not only the accuracy and precision of science, but the eloquence of poetry woven into each aphorism, right from Patanjali's *atha yoga anuśāsanam* (I.1) to *puruṣartha-śūnyānāṃ gunānāṃ pratiprasavaḥ kaivalyaṃ svarūpa-pratiṣṭhā vā citi-śaktir iti* (IV.34).

Those of you who are interested in a deep study of Raja Yoga will have to begin with the ten Upanishads—Isha, Kena, Katha, Prashna, Mundaka, Manduka, Taittiriya, Aitareya, Chandogya, Brihadaranyaka. I am suggesting this deep study only for those in the Western world who want to go through Raja Yoga or through the science of Yoga, dedicating their lives to it. If you have no time to study all of them, the Ishavasya Upanishad, Shvetashvatara Upanishad, Sixth Chapter of Gita, some parts of Yajnavalkya Smriti, Hatha Yoga Pradipika, and Patanjali's Raja Yoga can be studied. Those who are not interested in the personal transformation of consciousness, they need not read all that, but those who want to teach Raja Yoga, they would contribute quite a lot if they studied what was mentioned earlier.

Now let us come back to the sutra of this morning: *sattva-puruṣayoḥ śuddhi-sāmye kaivalyam-iti* (III.56).

Sattva—substance, *puruṣa*—the supreme intelligence, *śuddhi*—purity, *sāmye*—equal. Patanjali says that when the purity of *sattva,* that is, the matter *(prakṛti)* part of your being, is similar in quality to the purity of *puruṣa,* then that state of blended purity of *prakṛti* and *puruṣa* is called *kaivalyam.*

What is the matter part of your being? The sense organs. The mechanism of sensory perception has to be studied. The mechanism of mental perception—perception through word, through ideas, through thought—has to be studied.

For the purification of *sattva,* or the matter part of your being, you have to study how perception takes place and how cognizance takes place.

What are these sense organs? How do they come into contact with objects outside the skin? What happens to them? What is the quality of each sense organ—the glandular part, the muscular part, the part of the nervous system connected in the brain? How does the perception take place on the sensory level? What is the mechanism of sensory perception?

When one knows about that mechanism with the help of words, one begins to watch its functioning. One gets personally acquainted with its functioning, and then one understands the mechanism. Knowledge, acquaintance, and understanding—these are the three steps which one has to take in order that the purification of the mechanism takes place. Understanding will purify. We don't have to worry, How will I get purified? Purification is the by-product of clarity of understanding. Not knowledge that is verbal acquaintance. The verbal acquaintance is just opening the gate and entering the premises. There has to be verbal acquaintance and understanding taking place together.

In the same way, we will have to get acquainted with the mechanism of mind. What is the anatomy of thought? What is the chemistry of thought and mind? In order to understand the mechanism of mental perception, again we have to go through the same process. Acquire knowledge, that is, get verbally, intellectually acquainted, gather information, organize it, create an order in it, and then watch how the mind works. You get acquainted with the working of the mind, and that encounter with the fact of mental movement results in understanding.

Sattva śuddhi—the purification of the matter part—requires investigation through knowledge, investigation through observation, and then arriving at understanding.

If yoga students have only read books, gathered information, but have not observed practically the physical and mental mechanism, the quality of sensory and mental perception, how the perception takes place, what happens to the nerves and the chemical system when an emotion moves in the body, when a thought moves in the body, then it will be only sterile knowledge.

You have to work hard upon yourself—watching and observing. If one has not done it, then one will merely create purification at the physical level. The asanas, pranayama, and balanced nutrition will give better health and a beautiful, symmetrical, healthy body. That is also very important, that is the foundation, but is not one to proceed with it any further?

One is very much interested that the lovers of yoga in Europe and America do not stop at or get stuck at the physical part of yoga—asana, pranayama, *neti-dhauti,* etc., or perhaps *dhāraṇā*—and look upon yoga only as a therapy for physical health and physical beauty. Let them enrich their physical lives, but let them not look upon the science of yoga as meant only for balanced nutrition, curing sickness, etc. That would be touching only a hundredth part of yoga. That is only the introduction.

The purification of mental perception should be a concern of yoga teachers and yoga students. One feels Europe now is ready to proceed further. Observation of mental movement, understanding the whole anatomy and chemistry of thought and mind is the step that has to be taken. The study of *pratyāhāra* and *dhāraṇā* can help the purification of the mental body. We have to go up to purifying the *buddhi,* or intellect, which, according to Patanjali, is part of nature, part of *prakṛti.* Purification has to start from the sensory and culminate in the purification of *buddhi.* When that purification takes place, then for the crystallization or stabilization of the state of purification, meditation, or *dhyāna,* helps.

One has gone up to *dhāraṇā,* and let us suppose that one has arrived at the purification of mind and *buddhi,* or intellect. Then the six steps of meditation would be stabilized. The steadiness, the purification, the stabilization requires relaxation of activity. If you are moving, active, if you are experiencing then the stabilizing, the settling down, the metabolic relaxation cannot happen.

Meditation is a state when you are not moving anywhere. Consciously or voluntarily, you are not the doer, the knower, the experiencer. All movement has ended with *dhāraṇā,* and in *dhyāna* you are just at the source of your being—nondoing, nonknowing, nonexperiencing, noninvestigating, nonexploring. You know—just being. Because *puruṣa* has Beingness, creativity. It has a perception that is a nonmental, a noncerebral perception. It is a supramental or nonmental perception that Intelligence has, that the Supreme Intelligence of *puruṣa* has. The Supreme Understanding of *puruṣa* is something supramental, nonmental, nonsensory.

Unless one puts oneself, unless the whole *sattva,* the whole matter part of your being, is put into a state of unconditional relaxation, unconditional stillness, or Silence, unless there is a voluntary cessation of all movements from the sensory to the intellectual level, there cannot be the state of *dhyāna. Sattva* includes this whole realm of matter up to mind and intellect. So the movement has to cease in the whole of matter, in all the layers of matter. Mind and *buddhi* is the finest layer, and even their movement has to cease. *Manas,* or mind, is the collecting agency, and *buddhi* is the receiving, retaining, reproducing agent. *Buddhi* analyzes, discriminates, and, whenever needed, reproduces. All these agents, from receiving up to reproducing, have to cease moving.

Yama-niyama-āsana-prāṇāyāmā-pratyāhāra up to *dhāraṇā* are movements. Now there is the nondoing in order to purify. The purification gets stabilized in relaxation, as the health of the body stabilizes during sleep. You may eat the best food, do the best exercises in the world, but if you are unable to sleep, then there is no health, because whatever you had acquired throughout the day through nutrition, exercises, good thoughts, or whatever you call it, it has to stabilize, has to percolate to each level—chemical, neurological—to the whole metabolism, it has to percolate to each cell, to each drop of blood. That happens in sleep, therefore when you wake up in the morning you feel rejuvenated. Revitalization takes place in the state of meditation, or *dhyāna.*

When one has reached up to, when one has grown into, that state and cumulative purification has taken place, then there is *sattva-puruṣayoḥ śuddhi-sāmye*—assimilation in the quality of purification. The matter has been refined. The gross matter and fine matter, they have been refined through scientific education, through scientific conditioning, and the refinement has stabilized through meditation. Only then can the transformation in the quality of consciousness take place.

The gross energies and the finest possible aspect of matter—the energy part—have to be purified and stabilized. Even the energy of thought, the energy of intellect has to be purified, for it is still covered by matter. And then you come to understanding and awareness, which are the finest possible energies.

CHAPTER TWELVE

Indications of Samadhi

Tataḥ kleśa-karma-nivṛttiḥ (IV.30)

How do you know that a person has grown into the state of *kaivalyam* or is living in the state of *kaivalyam,* which is called *samādhi, mukti,* satori? How does one know? Are there any indications that the person really has now grown into the state of yoga, that he is a yogi? Teaching asana, pranayama, or *dhāraṇā* does not entitle you to call yourself a yogi. Unless one lives in the dimension of *samādhi,* and that dimension of *samādhi* is manifested in each movement—physical, verbal, psychological, cerebral, just as the *caitanya,* the Intelligence of the *puruṣa,* is manifested in the cosmos—then one cannot call oneself a yogi.

Patanjali refers to two indications. When there is that dimension of *samādhi,* there is *kleśa-karma-nivṛttiḥ,* that is, there is a total absence—*nivṛttiḥ*—there is total absence of *karma* or *kleśa* in the life of that person. That is to say, such a person who has arrived at the dimension of *samādhi* or has grown, has culminated, into the dimension of *samādhi,* he has no desire to earn or gain anything for himself or herself from the sensory, the mental, the nonmental movements taking place in his or her body or the movements taking place outside the body. He does not want anything from the world or from the purified states or the purified movements in the body. Do you see that these powers are not for exhibition, they are not for selling? He does not set up a shop or set up a sect or a dogma.

Karma-nivṛttiḥ—no motivation and no seeking anything for himself. Care is taken for the sustenance of the body, care is taken that the body is clothed properly, fed properly, but not because he would get some sensual pleasure from it. If that pleasure takes place, it is accepted; if it does not take place, it is accepted; if it does not take place, it is not sought. No denial, no seeking, no suppression, no asking. He does not want anything from his own body as a pleasure, he does not want anything from his knowledge or scholarship or erudition. No desire for name, fame, prestige, power, money. You see the definition of renunciation: when you do not want anything from the purification, attainments, achievements in your own body. They are not means to an end. So his movements are not the bargaining counters. No selling or purchasing or exhibiting. Living for the sake of living. Living for the joy of living, because the act of living is the only worship of the Divine. The act of living is the expression of gratitude toward *puruṣa*—the Supreme Intelligence.

He wants nothing outside life, nothing from life, nothing to obtain, nowhere to go, and yet the physical, the mental, the verbal, the movement in relationship is gone through with sensitivity, intelligence, love, and compassion. He does not want anything for himself, even from his own body, mind, or brain, because there is no *kleśa*. There is nothing like suffering in the being of that person.

When alone, when in the company of other people, in the day, in the night, in pain and in pleasure, in sickness, in health, in success, in failure, you will never find that the person is suffering. Psychological suffering has ended. It is only when you do not want anything from God or man, or from your own body or brain that suffering ends completely. Please do not forget that we have discriminated between psychological suffering and physical pain. Sickness there might be, even in the life of a yogi. Patanjali says only this: *kleṣah-nivṛttiḥ*. Psychological suffering has ended in such a person. And if it is not ended, then the person is not living in the state of *kaivalyam*. Look at the mathematical precision, look at the vast and deep implications when he talks about *kleśa* and *nivṛttiḥ, karma* and *nivṛttiḥ*.

That is why I wanted to talk with you this morning about *sattva-puruṣayoḥ śuddhi-sāmye kaivalyam-iti* (III.56). It may sound like Patanjali is talking about Utopia, but the great sage and seer has visualized the culmination of human growth in refinement, to this extent. After all, Divinity is nothing but refined humanity. If a human being goes on refining himself, at all the layers of his being, the essence of Divinity, which is unconditional love, compassion, intelligence, spontaneous understanding, etc., will begin to manifest through that human being. Divinity has to express itself through some form, and that person gets converted into the vehicle for the Supreme to manifest, to express. That is what a yogi is.

So Raja Yoga is a science of purification of perception, moderation of sense organs, and transformation in the human consciousness—three together, blended into one, which you call *jīvanyoga,* Yoga of Life. Just as there are Bhakti Yoga, Mantra Yoga, Tantra Yoga, Dhyana Yoga, and the Integral Yoga of Shri Aurobindo, the speaker has been using the term *jīvanyoga* for the Yoga of Life.

The Eastern world has had such yogis since the ancient days. Now the Western world, which is equipped with science and technology, with sufficient knowledge, and with an interest in yoga, could produce yogis or demonstrations of transformation in the content of consciousness. It seems to be the turn of the Western hemisphere. For a couple of centuries, Westerners have been interested in the study of the Vedas and Upanishads—they have translated them into German, French, English, and they have also written commentaries on them. In the last twenty-five years, the West has started taking an interest in yoga. A person like me feels hopeful that sincere and serious-minded students of yoga will take *pratyāhāra, dhāraṇā, dhyāna, samādhi*—the second part of Ashtanga Yoga—seriously. I hope that they won't stop at the first half—at the first four steps—but take seriously the second part and allow that mutation in the psyche to take place in their lives.

It was this hope that made me give consent to the suggestion that I spend some days with yoga teachers. I was anxious to have participants in the camp who have studied at least the theoretical part of Raja Yoga and have taught Hatha Yoga for five to ten years, so we could go deeper, not talk about the elementary, preliminary parts of the science of yoga, but explore and go as deep as it is possible to go with the help of words.

Appendix I: Sutras

Here is a list of the main sutras discussed in this book, along with translations compiled by editor Kaiser Irani.

Chapter 2
yogaś-citta-vṛtti-nirodhaḥ (I.2)
If consciousness *(citta)* is free *(nirodhaḥ)* from the ripples *(vṛtti)* of memory, only then yogic perception takes place.

Chapter 3
ahiṃsā-satya-asteya-brahmacarya-aparigrahā yamāḥ (II.30)
The yamas or universal principles of life are: not hurting oneself or others *(ahiṃsā);* discovering the truth for oneself *(satya);* not stealing or accepting unearned income *(asteya);* living the awareness of the ultimate reality *(brahmacarya);* non-attachment to possessions *(aparigrahā).*

Chapter 4
iti jāti-deśa-kāla-samaya-anavacchinnāḥ sārvabhaumā mahā-vratam (II.31)
The yamas are absolute values of life that are universally applicable *(sārvabhaumā),* irrespective of what race *(jāti)* you belong to, where you are *(deśa),* or what period of human history *(kāla)* you belong to; they are a choiceless acceptance (*mahā-vratam*) of the truth that one has perceived and understood.

Chapter 5
śauca-santoṣa-tapaḥ-svādhyāya-īśvara-praṇidhānāni niyamāḥ (II.32)
The niyamas or personal disciplines are: purity of the physical and psychophysical structure *(śauca);* contentment *(santoṣa);* austerity *(tapaḥ);* study *(svādhyāya);* feeling the presence *(praṇidhānā)* of the supreme Intelligence *(īśvara)* that surrounds you and is within you.

Chapter 6

tapaḥ svādhyāya īśvara-praṇidhānāni kriyāyogaḥ (II.1)

When every action *(kriyā)* of yours is born of austerity *(tapaḥ)*, self-observation *(svādhyāya)*, and the awareness *(praṇidhānā)* of Divinity *(īśvara)* within you, then your action results in the state of yoga.

Chapter 7

avidyā-asmitā-rāga-dveṣa-abhiniveśāḥ kleśāḥ (II.3)

The causes of psychological suffering *(kleśāḥ)* are: ignorance of one's own nature *(avidyā)*; identification with the conceptual structure *(asmitā)*; demand for the repetition of pleasure resulting in attachment *(rāga)*; aversion *(dveṣa)*; and desire to cling to the body *(abhiniveśāḥ)*.

Chapter 11

sattva-puruṣayoḥ śuddhi-sāmye kaivalyam-iti (III.56)

When the purity of the matter *(sattva)* part of your being is equal to *(sāmye)* the purity *(śuddhi)* of the Seer *(puruṣa)*, then that is the state of absolute unconditional freedom *(kaivalyam)*.

Chapter 12

tataḥ kleśa-karma-nivṛttiḥ (IV.30)

(In the state of *kaivalyam*) there is the total absence *(nivṛttiḥ)* of movement *(karma)* and psychological suffering *(kleśa)* in the life of the person.

Appendix II: Glossary

abhiniveśa	clinging to or obsession with the body
abhyāsa	practice, study
ācāra	behavior
ācārya	teaching
adhyātma	self-understanding
agni	fire
ahaṃkāra	I-consciousness, ego, sense of self
ahiṃsā	nonkilling, nonviolence
ākāśa	sky, space
ānanda	bliss
aṇḍa	egg
antara kumbhaka	retention of breath after inhalation
āpa	earth
aparigraha	nonattachment to possessions
araṇya	forest
āraṇyaka	of the forest
āsana	yoga pose or posture
asmitā	egotism, identification with the conceptual structure
āśrama	ashram, a place of relaxation
asteya	nonstealing
aśuddhi	impurity
ātma/ātman	self
avidyā	ignorance
bhoja	bark of the bhuja tree
bhuja	a variety of Indian tree

brahmacarya	dedication to the Divinity of Life
brahman	ultimate reality, the supreme Intelligence
brahmāṇḍam	the cosmic egg
buddhi	intellect
caitanya	the supreme Intelligence
cakra	an energy center in the body
car	to walk, move, live
caraiveti	be always moving
carya	way of living
cit/ citta	consciousness
dakṣinā	right side
darśana/darśanāni (pl)	philosophy, that which has been seen
dhāraṇā	concentration
dhyāna	meditation without method or technique
draṣṭā	seer, the principle of seeing
draṣṭṛ	seer
draṣṭuḥ	seeing and seeingness
dṛśya	that which is seen
dukham	pain, hurt, disagreeable sensation
dveṣa	aversion, hatred
hiraṇyagarbha	golden womb
indriya/indriyāni (pl)	sense organ(s)
īśate	permeates
īśvara	the supreme Intelligence or Divinity
īśvara-praṇidhāna	awareness of the Divinity around and within you
jīva/jīvāḥ	soul(s)
jīvanyoga	the yoga of life
jñāna	knowledge
jñānatatva	knowledge of the essence
kaivalyam	absolute freedom

karma	movement, action
karuṇā	compassion
kleśa	cause of affliction, psychological suffering
kriyāyoga	the yoga of action
kṛṣi	agriculture
madhyama mārga	the middle path
mahat	the great principle, first manifestation of matter
maitrī	friendliness
manas	mind
mānava samskṛta	a cultured human being
mātra	primary elements
māyā	illusion
muditā	joy
mukti	liberation
mūla avidyā	the root of ignorance
mūlādhāra	at the root of the spine
muni	sage
neti-dhauti	nasal cleansing
nirbīja	seedless
nirvicāra	without reflection
nirvitarka	without analysis
nivṛttiḥ	total absence
niyamaḥ/niyamāḥ (pl)	personal discipline(s)
nṛ	human being
nṛpati	king, prince, protector of human beings
pañca	five, fivefold
paramātman	cosmic self or soul
paramadraṣṭā	cosmic seer
paramapuruṣa	cosmic intelligence
pati	protector

patra	a leaf, a leaf for writing upon
prakṛti	all matter including the realm of energy
prāṇa	vital energy
prāṇāyāma	yogic breathing, expansion of vital energy
prāṇī	creatures
praṇidhāna	awareness, dedication
pratyāhāra	moderation, restraint of the senses
prīyate	she or he is satisfied or gratified
pṛthivī	cereals, grains
puraṃ	shell
puruṣa/puruṣah (pl)	knowledge, intelligence, understanding
purva	former, those who have gone before
rāga	attachment
rāja	kingly, royal, the prince
rajas	the faculty of activity
rajate	she or he rules, governs
ṛṣi	rishi, sage
sabīja	with seed
sādhana	practice
sahasrāra cakra	energy center at the crown of the head
samādhi	state of total absorption
saṃskāra/saṃskārāḥ (pl)	subliminal impressions(s)
saṃskṛti	culture
sāmye	equal
santoṣa	contentment
sārvabhaumā	universal
sarvam dukham, sarvam śānikam	all is pain, all is fleeting
sat	truth
satta	to-be-ness
sattva	substance, the matter part of being
satya	truthfulness

śauca	purification
śavāsana	corpse pose
savicāra	with reflection
savitarka	with analysis
smṛti	memory, recollection
śram	exhaustion
śuddhi	pure
śuddhi-karaṇa	purification
sukham	happiness, agreeable sensation
sūri	wise man, seer
svādhyāya	study
tamas	the potential for inertia
tapas	austerity
tattva	an element or elementary property
upekṣā	non-attachment
vāma	left side
varaṇam	selection or choosing
vāyu	wind, vital airs
vid	to know
veda	the product of knowledge
vedānta	the ending of knowledge
vidyā	self-knowledge
virata	ceased, desisting from, ended
vratam	vow, choiceless acceptance
vrīyate	a choiceless acceptance
vṛtti	ripples, movement of thought
vyakti	individual
yama	universal principle of life
yoga	the art and science of joining and combining
yuj	to combine, join, blend
yujyate	she or he is joined with, yoked with

About the Author

Born in India, Vimala Thakar began her spiritual search at the tender age of five. As a young woman, she traveled and lectured for the Land Gift Movment of Vonoba Bhave, an associate of Mahatma Ghandi. Her meetings with Krishnmurti, from 1956 to 1961, had a profound effect on her life. From the 1960s to the 1980s, she taught meditation retreats in thirty-five countries. She stopped traveling outside India in 1991, and now resides in Mount Abu, in Rajastan, where she meets with people from all over the world.

Rodmell Press published her *Blossoms of Friendship,* which launched the Yoga Wisdom Classics series.

From the Publisher

Shambhala Publications is pleased to publish the Rodmell Press collection of books on yoga, Buddhism, and aikido. As was the aspiration of the founders of Rodmell Press, it is our hope that these books will help individuals develop a more skillful practice—one that brings peace to their daily lives and to the Earth.

To learn more, please visit www.shambhala.com.

Index

yama of, described, 21–22
ātman (Self), 64. *See also puruṣa* (Cosmic Self)
attachment. *See rāga*
Aurobindo's Integral Yoga, 88–89
austerity. *See tapas*
aversion *(dveṣa)*, 46, 80. *See also* kleshas *(kleśa)*
avidyā (ignorance). *See also* kleshas *(kleśa)*
as clouded perception by the Seer, 66, 71–72
freedom from, 77–78
klesha described, 41–43
letting go of, 84
origin of, 67
avidyā-asmitā-rāga-dveṣa-abhiniveśāḥ kleśāḥ (II.3), 39–51, 80, 98. *See also* kleshas *(kleśa)*

body
educating in steadiness, 13–14
freeing from conditionings, 28
identification with, 42
obsession with *(abhiniveśa)*, 46–47, 79–80
purifying sense organs through *tapas*, 32–34
brahmacarya (dedication to the Divinity of Life). *See also* yamas
as an absolute value, 23, 25
choiceless acceptance of *(mahā-vratam)*, 26
as demonstration of awareness of unity, 20
klesha described, 22–23
as universal *(sārvabhaumā)*, 21, 24, 25–26
Brahman, 22
brain
educating to be free of movement, 14–15
purifying through study *(svādhyāya)*, 35–36
buddhi (intellect)
cessation of movement in, 92
defined, 72, 92
interpretation by, 66
mind *(manas* or *citta)* versus, 64
purification of, 91
thinking and, 72

carya (way of living), 22
celibacy versus *brahmacarya*, 23
chakras *(cakra)*, Tantra Yoga and, 55–56
change
constancy of, 78, 79
freedom from attachment *(rāga)* and, 78–79
thought structure or thought stream and, 79–80
choiceless acceptance *(vratam)*, 26
citta (mind), 64, 72
clarity versus purification, 35–36
clinging to the body *(abhiniveśa)*, 46–47, 79–80. *See also* kleshas *(kleśa)*
Communism, 22
concentration. *See dhāraṇā*
conditioning
culture and, 4, 53–56
defined, 4
dhāraṇā (concentration) and, 53–54, 56–60, 84
educating the body to be free of, 28
in pranayama, 55
of the senses, 32
in Tantra Yoga, 55–56
contentment *(santoṣa)*, 27
corruption, 21–22
Cosmic Self. *See puruṣa*
cosmos, created from *puruṣa*, 68–69, 75–76

creativity, energy of
process of manifestation, 75–76
self-aware in humans, 77
shared by matter, 76
culture *(saṃskṛti)*, as result of conditionings, 4–5

dark night of the soul, 50
darśana (to see), 71
darśanāni (Darshan philosophy), 71
dedication to the Divinity of Life. *See brahmacarya*
dhāraṇā (concentration), 53–60
art of living and, 83–84
conditioning and, 53–54, 56–60, 84
dhyāna (meditation) versus, 60
latent powers developed by, 59–60
methods and techniques, 57–59
moderation toward mind learned by, 83–84
as necessary for *dhyāna* (meditation), 62
progression of practices up to, 59
dhyāna (meditation)
art of living and, 84–85
dhāraṇā (concentration) and, 60, 62
as effortless, 62
as ending of movement, 61, 91–92
inertia or passivity versus, 62
methods and techniques ended by, 61, 62
discipline, 32–34. *See also tapas* (austerity)
Divinity, feeling the presence of. *See īśvara praṇidhāna*
Divinity of life, dedication to. *See brahmacarya*
draṣṭā dṛśi-mātraḥ śuddho'pi pratyaya-anupaśyaḥ (II.20), 64, 66–67, 69
draṣṭā (Seer). *See also puruṣa* (Cosmic Self)
avidyā (ignorance) as clouded perception by, 66, 67, 71–72
contact between seen and, 65–66
defined, 64
identification with the seen, 66–67, 71–72
individual and, 70
not the doer, 64–65
puruṣa (Cosmic Self) as, 71
draṣṭṛ dṛśyayoḥ saṃyogo heya-hetuḥ (II.17), 64
dṛśya (seen), 65–66, 68
duḥkhānuśayī dveśaḥ (II.8), 45, 46
dukham (disagreeable sensation), 40, 46
dveṣa (aversion), 46, 80. *See also* kleshas *(kleśa)*

earth *(pṛthivī)*, 76
ecology, 17
educating
body in steadiness, 13–14
body to be free of conditionings, 28
brain to be free of movement, 14–15
for purifying the body, 33
through repetition *(abhyāsa)*, 54, 84
training versus, 54–55
egoism *(asmitā)*, 43–45. *See also* kleshas *(kleśa)*
energy
conserved through moderation *(pratyāhāra)*, 83
of creativity, 75–76, 77
creativity shared by matter, 76
prāṇa (vital energy), 75
purification of, 92
thought as energy in matter, 76–77
world as field of, 77
Engels, Friedrich, 22

experiences, self-discovery through, 78–79
eyes, closing, 14

farm culture *(kṛṣi saṃskṛti)*, 5–6
feeling *(praṇidhāna)*, 29–30, 38
feeling the presence of Divinity. *See īśvara praṇidhāna*
fire *(agni)*, 75
fivefold kleshas *(pañca kleśaḥ)*. *See* kleshas *(kleśa)*
forest culture *(āraṇyaka saṃskṛti)*, 3
freedom
  from attachment *(rāga)*, 78–79
  from conditionings, 28
  from ignorance *(avidyā)*, 77–78
  kaivalyam as absolute freedom, 88
  from obsession with the body *(abhiniveśa)*, 79–80
  from suffering *(kleśa)*, 47–51
  from thinking, 14–15, 16–17

glossary, 99–103
great choiceless acceptance *(mahā-vratam)*, 26
ground of existence, 87

harmony, 19–20, 80–81
history. *See* Vedic period
holistic way of living
  Raja Yoga as, 8, 10
  in Vedic period, 7–8, 9
  yamas as, 26
humility as expression of *praṇidhāna*, 38

ideational knowledge, 15–16, 43, 44
identification
  with the body, 42
  of the Seer with the seen, 66–67, 71–72
ignorance. *See avidyā*
indriya. *See* sense organs
I-ness or Me-ness
  asmitā (egoism), 43–45
  functioning from, without self-centeredness, 38
  as an idea, 16, 43
  identification of the Seer with, 66–67, 71–72
  kleshas (suffering) as creation of, 50
Integral Yoga of Shri Aurobindo, 88–89
intellect. *See buddhi*
Is-ness, 42
īśvara (all-permeating principle of Supreme Intelligence)
  dance of life and, 37–38
  defined, 29
  Patanjali's use of, 36–37
īśvara praṇidhāna (feeling the presence of Divinity)
  as attitude of surrender, 37–38
  īśvara, 29, 36–38
  niyama, 29–30
  praṇidhāna, 29–30, 38
  sutra explaining, 32, 36–38
iti jāti-deśa-kāla-samaya-anavacchinnāḥ sārvabhaumā mahā-vratam (II.31), 25–26, 97. *See also* yamas

jīvanyoga (Yoga of Life), 95

kaivalyam, 88, 89, 93. *See also samādhi*
Kapila. *See* Samkhya of Kapila
karma-nivṛttiḥ (absence of karma), 93–94
kāya-indriya-siddhir aśuddhi-kṣayāt tapasaḥ (II.43), 32–34
kings or princes *(nṛpati)*, 6
kleśa-karma-nivṛttiḥ (absence of karma and klesha), 93

Patanjali Yoga as science of, 31
of perception through understanding, 89–90, 91
of perception, to see the truth, 26
pratyāhāra (moderation) and, 82–83
ṛṣyo mantradṛṣṭāro (purified perception), 3
samādhi and, 82
sattva-puruṣayoḥ śuddhi-sāmye (assimilation in the quality of purification), 92
sattva-śuddhi (purification of matter), 90–91
of sense organs, 89–90
tapas (austerity) for the sake of, 32–34
purified perception *(ṛṣyo mantradṛṣṭāro)*, 3
puruṣa (Cosmic Self), 63–73. *See also* *draṣṭā* (Seer)
ākāśa manifested from, 75
awareness of, as destiny of man, 84
contact between Seer and seen, 65–66
cosmos created from, 68–69, 75–76
as *draṣṭā* (Seer), 71
duality with *prakṛti*, 70–71
as ground of existence, 87
inbuilt quality of perception or understanding, 69
independent from *prakṛti* (nature or matter), 64, 65
individual *puruṣāḥ*, 69–70
mahat manifested from, 75
not the doer, 64–65
other terms for, 64, 70
prakṛti (nature or matter) as opportunity to experience, 65
in Samkhya of Kapila, 63–64
yoga as discrimination between *prakṛti* and, 67–69
rāga (attachment). *See also* kleshas *(kleśa)*
aparigraha (nonpossessiveness) versus, 24
freedom from, 78–79
klesha described, 45–46
as suffering, 80
rāga-dveṣa. *See dveṣa* (aversion); *rāga* (attachment)
Rāja (prince), 10
relationships
obsession with the body *(abhiniveśa)* and, 47
as test for validity of truth, 2
repulsion *(dveṣa)*, 46, 80. *See also* kleshas *(kleśa)*
rishis
attributes of, 3
derivation of the term, 3
homes as *āśrama*, 6–7
ṛṣi saṃskṛti (rishi culture), 3–5
sages as incomplete meaning for, 3
ṛṣi (purified perception), 3. *See also* rishis
ṛṣi saṃskṛti (rishi culture), 3–5
ṛṣyo mantradṛṣṭāro (purified perception), 3

sages, rishis as better term for, 3
samādhi
as culmination of Ashtanga Yoga, 88
elimination of impurities and, 82
as freedom from suffering, 85
growth into dimension of, 84
indications of, 93–95
kinds and qualities of, 61–62
kleśa-karma-nivṛttiḥ (absence of karma and klesha) in, 93–94
as living in the state of *kaivalyam*, 93

training
  educating versus, 54–55
  for purifying the body, 33–34
truth, relationships as test for validity of, 2
truthfulness. *See satya*

understanding. *See also puruṣa* (Cosmic Self)
  adhyātma (self-understanding), 41
  purifying sense organs through, 89–90
  as purpose of human life, 78
  sattva-śuddhi (purification of matter) through, 90–91
  self-awareness enabling, 77
universal *(sārvabhaumā)*, yamas as, 21, 25–26

vedānta, 2
Vedas, 2–3
Vedic period
  āraṇyaka saṃskṛti (forest culture), 3
  āśrama saṃskṛti (ashram culture), 6–9
  discoveries of, 11
  holistic way of living in, 7–8, 9
  kṛṣi saṃskṛti (farm culture), 5–6
  record of verbal communications in, 2
  ṛṣi saṃskṛti (rishi culture), 3–5
vid (to know), 2
vidyā (self-knowledge), 41, 43
vital energy *(prāṇa)*, 75
"vow" *(vratam)*, 26
vṛtti (thought movement), 17. *See also* thinking

water *(āpa)*, 75–76

yamas
  as absolute values, 23, 25
  ahiṃsā (nonviolence or nonkilling), 19–20
  aparigraha (nonpossessiveness), 23–24
  asteya (nonstealing), 21–22
  brahmacarya (dedication to the Divinity of Life), 20, 22–23
  choiceless acceptance of *(mahāvratam)*, 26
  harmonious living and, 80
  as holistic way of living, 26
  niyamas versus, 21
  satya (truthfulness), 20–21
  as universal *(sārvabhaumā)*, 21, 24, 25–26
yoga
  branches of, 10
  defined, 9–10
  derivation of the term, 9
  extending beyond Patanjali's sutras, 1
  going beyond the physical part, 91
  of Life, 95
yogaś-citta-vṛtti-nirodhaḥ (I.2), 13–17, 97

Printed in the United States
by Baker & Taylor Publisher Services